Exploring Rituals in Nursing

Zane Robinson Wolf, PhD, RN, FAAN is dean emerita and professor, School of Nursing and Health Sciences at La Salle University, and returned to full-time teaching in the fall of 2012. Her courses include nursing research, patient safety, evidence-based practice, and caring, and she continues to conduct qualitative and quantitative research on medication errors, nurse caring, nursing education concerns, and other topics. Dr. Wolf practiced as a critical care and medical-surgical nurse and has worked in nursing education, teaching in diploma, associate, baccalaureate, master's, and doctoral nursing programs and was also the associate director of Nursing for Research at Einstein Healthcare System. Dr. Wolf is a board member of the Institute for Safe Medication Practices and a member of the patient safety committees of St. Christopher's Hospital for Children and Fox Chase Cancer Center. She is a board member of the Pennsylvania State Nurses Association and also reviews manuscripts for various nursing and health care journals. Dr. Wolf has been an editor of the *International Journal for Human Caring* since 1999 and a former board member and past president of the International Association for Human Caring having hosted three International Caring Conferences in Philadelphia. The Christine E. Lynn College of Nursing at Florida Atlantic University honored her by designating her a "caring scholar" and is a member of the Anne Boykin Institute for the Advancement of Caring in Nursing.

Exploring Rituals in Nursing

Joining Art and Science

Zane Robinson Wolf, *PhD, RN, FAAN*

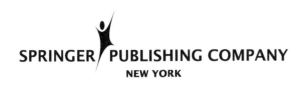

SPRINGER PUBLISHING COMPANY
NEW YORK

Watson Caring
Science Institute

Springer Publishing Company, LLC
11 West 42nd Street
New York, NY 10036
www.springerpub.com

Acquisitions Editor: Elizabeth Nieginski
Composition: Exeter Premedia Services Private Ltd.

ISBN: 978-0-8261-9662-0
e-book ISBN: 978-0-8261-9663-7

13 14 15 16 17/ 5 4 3 2 1

The author and the publisher of this Work have made every effort to use sources believed to be reliable to provide information that is accurate and compatible with the standards generally accepted at the time of publication. The author and publisher shall not be liable for any special, consequential, or exemplary damages resulting, in whole or in part, from the readers' use of, or reliance on, the information contained in this book. The publisher has no responsibility for the persistence or accuracy of URLs for external or third-party Internet websites referred to in this publication and does not guarantee that any content on such websites is, or will remain, accurate or appropriate.

Library of Congress Cataloging-in-Publication Data
Wolf, Zane Robinson.
Exploring rituals in nursing : joining art and science / Zane Robinson Wolf.
    p. ; cm.
  Includes bibliographical references.
  ISBN 978-0-8261-9662-0 – ISBN 978-0-8261-9663-7 (e-book)
  I. Title.
  [DNLM: 1. Nursing Process. 2. Ceremonial Behavior. 3. Interpersonal Relations. WY 100.1]
  RT41
  610.73–dc23

                                                                            2013015354

Printed in the United States of America by Courier.

I would like to thank my husband, Charles J. Wolf, MD, and colleagues at the School of Nursing and Health Science at La Salle University for their steadfast support. I also appreciate the ongoing support of the Christian Brothers of La Salle University and the blessings of my fall 2012 sabbatical. The staff at Springer Publishing Company have guided and encouraged me throughout this endeavor, including Elizabeth Nieginski, Chris Teja, and Alan Graubard, formerly of Springer. I am grateful for all that I have learned from my undergraduate, graduate, and doctoral nursing students.

This book is dedicated to the nurses and women in my life who have encouraged and sustained me. The art included in this book was found in the nursing journal, *The Trained Nurse*, that was subsequently named *The Trained Nurse and Hospital Review*. The art was published before 1900.

Zana Ellen Robinson
Gale Robinson-Smith, PhD, RN
Elise Robinson Pizzi, MSN, CRNP
Jessica Wolf Dasher, MPH
Ciara Anne Dasher
Rory Ellen Dasher
Zana Cecelia Wolf, MS, MBA
Leslie Robinson Jarrell, MD
Gwynneth Leslie Jarrell, BSN, RN
Azadeh Khodabandelou Jarrell, BS, RDMS
Kelly Jo Gastley Wolf, JD
Elizabeth Celia Wolf
Keven Mara Robinson, MD
Nicole Albano Robinson, BA
Lindsay Jones Pizzi, BA
Julia Peoples Robinson, MD
Nora Leslie Robinson, BS
Kerry Cornforth Robinson
Elaine Beldyk Siebold, BSN, RN
Sharon Creamer Murphy, RN
Patricia DiVello Ford
Kathleen Harrigan Czekanski, PhD, RN, CNE
Barbara J. Hoerst, PhD, RN
Denise Nagle Bailey, EdD, MEd, MSN, RN, CSN
Mary T. Dorr, MSN, RN
Karen Rossi, MSN, RN, ACNS-BC
Patti Rager Zuzelo, EdD, RN, ACNS-BC, ANP-BC, FAAN
Sister Rose Carmel Scalone, EdD, MPH, BSN, RSM
Anne Boykin, PhD, RN
Kathleen Valentine, PhD, RN
Marian Turkel, PhD, RN, NEA-BC, FAAN
Renee C. Fox, PhD
Jean Watson, PhD, RN, AHN-BC, FAAN

CONTENTS

FOREWORD

It has been noted that we need a revolution of rituals in our world today: the world that now presents us with disconnections, discontinuous and asynchronous communication and relationships; separation of meaning from experiences; transcendence of time, space, and physicality; and no distinction between data and information, information from knowledge. We are often left bereft with little or no understanding and no space or place for wisdom. Nursing rituals offer a human reprieve and refuge that helps us unite, tying together our separate parts reconciling the sacred and the profane, the intimate with the cold impersonal, offering a ground of purposive action in an otherwise abyss of human and clinical, professional and scientific, technical complexities.

Zane Wolf is an expert in translating and grounding theory and abstracts into understanding and revealing critical practical rituals that stabilize us and our practice world; she helps us to integrate the personal with the professional.

Through Dr. Wolf's comprehensive approach to helping us understand and integrate rituals, we recognize clinical rituals as important pointers that translate theory into purposeful, intentional, conscious art acts. Rituals serve as critical reminders, as anchors of personal intimate experiences and actions. Rituals serve as ceremonial acts, as turning points for celebration, or as guiding actions of passages of time and life moments. When we integrate rituals and understanding of purposeful rituals into our life and our clinical practice, we allow for smooth and purposeful life processes and transitions. Rituals help us to let go, opening to new, passing certain thresholds of life experiences, traumas as well as traditions.

Rituals in nursing are memory making, giving new directions for concrete practices. This book examines ritualistic meanings, symbolic interpretations, along with the overall role rituals play in an otherwise chaotic world of care.

Nursing rituals continue to be performed as timeless acts that stabilize the complexities of tumultuous care. They remain in the private inner world of nursing care, serving significant and important symbolic functions to honor and sustain basic human care needs at personal, professional, social, and cultural levels, providing respites in the midst of an otherwise impersonal institutional darkness.

Rituals comingle with science and theory. They provide an inner private intimacy to the impersonal, often cold and detached professional clinical gaze of health and sick care, of birthing and dying practices. Nursing rituals take place in nurse-to-patient, human-to-human intimate care moments and personal situations. Dr. Wolf's work highlights the sacred and profane nature of nursing.

This updated, scholarly, and wise view of classic nursing rituals incorporates theory with evidence-based research. The structure of the book moves from the background of the importance of rituals, to exploring the interpersonal artistic expression of rituals via several caring theories, for example, Paterson and Zderad; Watson, Boykin, and Schoenhofer; and Halldorsdottir.

This comprehensive text captures the vast nursing rituals and their traditions; such commonalities as bathing; bodywork; postmortem care; medications administration including rituals of safety and error prevention; and notions of confession, disclosure, and reporting of errors, all highly ritualized in their function and purpose.

Other rituals are identified and uncovered, such as socialization into the profession, and rites of passage are identified, named, and explored for us as the reader learns to be more cognizant and conscious of how we use ceremonial rituals. We have rituals for entrance into the profession, its traditions, beliefs, and customs, often taken for granted, but not illuminated.

And finally, in a most updated social and professional view of nursing rituals, this book helps us celebrate our own ceremonies across time such as capping, pinning, senior programs, and nurse practitioner ceremonies. However, the most interesting final touch is recognizing national ritualistic ceremonies such as the celebration of National Nurses Week and nurses' work and scholarship, highlighted by American Academy of Nursing's induction ceremony. This ceremony is perhaps the pinnacle of a mature discipline and profession for the ancient and timeless, yet very contemporary, profession of nursing. This mature and evolving profession of nursing, in the end, with all its transition and change, lives by ritual.

This work helps us to critique, to awaken to our history, our traditions, and our gifts to sustain human intimacy and professional practice we can recognize and intentionally integrate. Through this deeper understanding and uncovering of rituals, we can more fully celebrate the beauty of concrete nursing rituals that keep us whole and holy, even in the midst of the profane.

I am honored and privileged to participate in the ritual of endorsing this special scholarly work as a collection in Watson Caring Science–Springer Caring Science Library collection. This ritual practice and publication of the Caring Science Library will keep alive classic and timeless caring science literature for past and future generations. This work is one of them.

Jean Watson, PhD, RN, AHN-BC, FAAN
Founder/Director Watson Caring Science Institute
Distinguished Professor and Dean Emerita
University of Colorado Denver, College of Nursing
www.watsoncaringscience.org

PREFACE

Rituals in Nursing examines nursing as a cultural system through purposeful reflection on selected nursing rituals. Almost inadvertently, the book brings nursing issues, trends, and roles into focus. It is a reexamination of nursing rituals in the context of professional nursing practice and continues my fascination with the topic that began with my dissertation at the School of Nursing at the University of Pennsylvania. An implicit subtext throughout the book is my conviction that nurse caring is essential to patients, families, and colleague nurses. As a reexamination of rituals in nursing, the chapters in the book bring forth some of the hidden, symbolic meanings of nurses' work.

Nursing rituals take place in daily nursing practice. They serve many important functions, both practical and social, and distinguish the culture of nursing as some of its more private, hidden work is carried out. Nursing rituals take place in nurse-to-patient, direct care situations and in nurse-to-nurse situations, and mark transitions into the professional nursing role. Rituals show the sacred and profane of nursing through their performance.

Similar to Taylor (1994), I believe that nursing operates in social contexts in which intersubjective meanings are generated and are crucial to the healing of patients and nurses. In the many settings in which nursing care is provided, there are nursing rituals that are performed. They do not replace science, but coexist with it. Consequently, arguers deriding rituals might take another look, perhaps using the lenses of nursing, anthropology, and sociology.

Rituals in nursing, including nursing practice and socialization rituals, demonstrate nurses' commitment to patients and families and to one another. The orientation of the rituals in caring–healing for patients, families, and fellow nurses is rooted in the essential ethical values of beneficence and respect for human dignity. As such, they operationalize nursing's commitment to "touch the human center of the person" (Watson, 1988, p. 176) by the genuine intention to do good and value the worth and integrity of all humans through compassionate care. Rituals help nurses transcend moments and potentiate healing. Those involved in transpersonal caring moments are consequently restored and preserved as they experience the health care system as mutual recipients and providers of caring and healing (Watson, 1988). Compassionate human service sustains and preserves human dignity and is deeply concerned with relationships between caregivers and care recipients (Clarke, Watson, & Brewer, 2009).

The prologue, "Rituals in Nursing: Underpinnings and Importance," lays the foundation for the book. Definitions and descriptions of rituals are presented from the vantage points of different disciplines. The elements of rituals are emphasized with how they appear during ritual performances. Nursing literature on ritual is followed by positive and negative perspectives of nurse scholars. Section I, "Rituals of Nursing Practice," concentrates on examples from daily nursing work. The interpersonal caring ritual and interpersonal relationships, bathing patients as a ritual in transition, postmortem care, and ritualistic prevention of medication errors are deliberately reviewed from the organizing themes of tradition and procedures, initiation into ritual performance, evolving research, art and ritual, and ritual symbols.

Section II, "Rituals of Socialization," addresses change-of-shift reports and nursing ceremonies. These examples mark the transitions into professional nursing and some of the celebrations of professional nursing work in health care agencies. Initiation into the role of the nurse through change-of-shift reports and types of ceremonies are described along with related research and ritual symbols. Finally, the Epilogue provides a classification of the rituals in nursing investigated in this book and points out the ethical values at their foundation.

This book originates in the reflections and perspectives of a nurse–academic who values the enormous contribution of direct care registered nurses at the front line and at the sharp end of health care delivery. It is then an integration of thoughts, beliefs, values, and literature. Because of this, the strengths and limitations of the work are mine.

Zane Robinson Wolf, PhD, RN, FAAN

PROLOGUE

Rituals in Nursing: Underpinnings and Importance

Rituals coexist in American nursing culture along with many other aspects of the profession, for example, beliefs about the profession, use of technology, and application of science to clinical practice. How nursing rituals and rituals in nursing intermingle with cultural norms, customs, routines, art, technology, and science is important to understand. It is also worthwhile to clarify the meanings, persistence, elimination, and transformation of rituals. Nursing rituals may show that nurses are carrying out a developing international resurgence in reclaiming nursing as a profession (Ferguson et al., 2008; Hales, 2003).

In spite of laudable, essential, and critical efforts aimed at underpinning professional practice with evidence, science fails to answer all of the problems of clinical nursing work. Because of this, rituals are worth exploring. Nonetheless, nursing rituals and ritualism have been scrutinized in nursing literature for decades and not always appreciated in the context of viewing nursing as a cultural group. This attention, while sometimes controversial, signifies their importance and the value of examining this aspect of the culture of the nursing profession. In addition, some rituals incorporate both the sacred and profane of nursing work.

The nursing profession's rituals provide an expressive and powerful supplement to its beliefs, art, and science. Nursing owns its rituals in the same way that the profession has a distinctive culture. Nursing rituals demonstrate patterns of cultural behavior that assist in transmitting traditional knowledge and practices. They help nurses maintain social order by cohesion and interaction (Suominen, Kovasin, & Ketola, 1997). This book explores ritual definitions from the lenses of various disciplines, analyzes ritual elements and symbols, and examines themes pertaining to rituals in nursing literature.

RITUAL FOUNDATIONS, DEFINITIONS, AND ELEMENTS

Many cultural groups perform rituals that distinguish their social interactions and partially shape their identities. According to classic anthropological thought, rituals arise from crises of human existence, for example, those taking place during the circumstances of conception, pregnancy, birth, puberty, marriage, and death (Malinowski, 1992). Rituals are part of the fabric of human existence and accompany beliefs and rites. Often they combine with beliefs, religion, and magic, particularly surrounding the beginning and end of life.

For example, Malinowski asserted that:

During pregnancy the expectant mother has to keep certain taboos and undergo ceremonies, and her husband shares at times in both. At birth, before and after, there are various magical rites to prevent dangers and undo sorcery, ceremonies of purification, communal rejoicings, and acts of presentation of the newborn to higher powers or to the community. (1992, p. 37)

As death approaches, the nearest relatives in any case, sometimes the whole community, forgather by the dying man, and dying, the most private act which a man can perform, is transformed into a public, tribal event. (1992, p. 48)

Rituals are sometimes defined as practices that reflect relief of anxiety through performance of repetitive or obsessionally precise symbolic acts. Compulsive gestures, repetitive behaviors, and mechanical praying are also listed as elements of ritual (Murdock et al., 1961). Rituals contain a high level of symbolic activity and involve a degree of formality, rigidity, simplicity of movement, repetitiveness, and rhythm (Davis, 1981). They express symbolic meanings important to groups of people functioning within a culture or subculture.

Rites of passage (van Gennep, 1960) are rituals attached to transitions in individuals' lives, such as marriage, purification after childbirth, and funerals after death. They are ceremonial, transitional rites including rites of separation, transition rites, and rites of incorporation. Preliminal rites are rites of separation; liminal rites are rites of transition; and postliminal rites are rites of incorporation (van Gennep, 1960). Liminality refers to thresholds.

TABLE P.1

Ritual Descriptions and Definitions Across the Disciplines

Definitions and Descriptions	Discipline	Citation
Ritual is prescribed formal behavior for occasions not given over to technological routine, having reference to mystical beings or powers. Ritual affirms communal unity.	Anthropology	Turner (1967, p. 19)
Rituals are dramas of social events that emphasize the importance of the event they symbolize or represent; they are standardized, repetitive dramatizations of social crises, functioning to minimize the effects of crisis. Rituals confront the individuals of the tribe with common values; ritual is drama symbolizing an important social event.		
Ritual is consecrated behavior; religious ritual involves symbolic fusion of ethos and world views. It involves a broad range of moods and motivations and metaphysical conceptions that shape the spiritual consciousness of a people; they are full-blown ceremonies as cultural performances. The symbolic acts of rituals are given order and structure by the explicitly stated purposes of those rituals.	Anthropology	Geertz (1973, pp. 34, 112–113)
[Ritual is] a generalized medium of social interaction in which the vehicles for constructing messages are iconic symbols (acts, words, or things) that convert the load of significance or complex sociocultural meanings embedded in and generated by the ongoing processes of social existence into a communication currency. …Shared sociocultural meanings constitute the utilities that are symbolically transacted through the medium of ritual action.	Social and cultural anthropology	Munn (1973, p. 580)
Rituals represent a passage from one position, constellation, or domain of structure to another and insure maintenance of a cosmic order which transcends the contradictions and conflicts inherent in the mundane social system. Rituals use symbolic objects and cyclical and repetitive activities.	Anthropology	Turner (1974, pp. 238, 249)
Public ritual expresses a common, public concern, and uses whatever symbolic language…for bringing the point home. Social context is important.	Anthropology	Douglas (1975, p. 67)
Ritual is patterned, symbolic action that refers to the goals and values of a social group.	Sociology	DeCraemer, Vansina, and Fox (1976, p. 469)
Ritual provides relief from anxiety both for sick individuals themselves and for others concerned with their welfare. Effective meaning of any ritual depends not only on the character of the ritual itself but also on the perspective from which it is viewed. Ritual relieves distress by making illness meaningful. When the study of ritual is linked to the study	Anthropology	McCreery (1979, pp. 53, 57, 69)

(continued)

TABLE P.1

Ritual Descriptions and Definitions Across the Disciplines (continued)

Definitions and Descriptions	Discipline	Citation
of healing, the therapeutic value of a ritual for particular individuals with particular problems becomes an issue of central importance. Behaviors, social, and cultural milieu, meanings, communication, and barriers to communication are important.... First, by working with knowledgeable informants, observing the behavior of participants in a ritual, and analyzing the social and cultural milieu in which it occurs, determines as far as possible what a ritual might mean. Second, consider the situation in which the ritual is observed and ask which of the ritual's possible meanings are relevant and which are not. Third, ask what means of communication and barriers to communication are actually operating in that situation. Rituals are symbolic constructions analogous to works of art or literature; they label problematic situations, articulate their internal organization and relationship to the world at large, and orient responses to them.	Sociology of medicine	Bosk (1980, pp. 71–72)
Occupational rituals, such as attending and work rounds, case conferences, grand rounds, and mortality and morbidity conferences, may be analyzed as occupational rituals that allow physicians to dramatize, to teach, and to remind themselves and their colleagues of their sense of what it means to be a physician. Occupational rituals help physicians to resolve social problems endemic to patient management: managing uncertainty, making treatment decisions, and evaluating outcomes.		
Rules that guide behaviors in corporate life and are dramatizations of a company's basic cultural values. Behind each ritual is a myth symbolizing a belief central to the culture.	Business	Deal and Kennedy (1982, p. 62)
Standardized, detailed set of techniques and behaviors that manages anxieties but seldom produces intended, practical consequences of any importance.	Business	Beyer and Trice (1987)

Definition	Discipline	Citation
Ritual is a significant feature of social life in that it secures a collective, extra-individual sense of events. Its patterned sequences are highly symbolic and thus meaningful for all participants, both actors and observers. The timing and order of events as well as role and identity of the participants carries condensed, symbolic information for those involved.	Anthropology	Sankar citing Rappaport (1991, p. 44)
Ritual has a prominent role in securing cultural knowledge; ritual is an eminently suitable device for organizing a theoretical conversation that wishes to uncover cultural meanings through the interpretation of texts.	Religion	Bell (1992, p. 54)
A ritual is a patterned, repetitive, and symbolic enactment of a cultural belief or value; its primary purpose is transformation.	Cultural anthropology	Davis-Floyd (1992, p. 19)
Rituals are visible expressions of community bonding and support through biological and psychological passages of life… the ways all societies give meaning, richness, and structure to life…rites of separation from old ways of being and thinking and behaving, and integrating into new modes of being.	Nursing	Achterberg, Dossey, & Kolkmeier (1994, p. 2)
Ritual connotes an already known, richly symbolic pattern of behavior, the emphasis falling less upon the making and more upon the valued pattern and its panoply of associations. …Ritual is vital in processes of social change.	Religion, theology	Driver (1998, p. 30)
Ritualizing denotes the activity of deliberately cultivating or inventing rites (specific enactments located in concrete times and places; often named and intentionally practiced) that are recognized by group consensus and are nonutilitarian and expressive.	Religion and culture	Grimes (2000, p. 29)

As dramas of social events, rituals emphasize the importance of the events they symbolize or represent. Turner (1967), an anthropologist, considered rituals as dramatizations of social crises that function to minimize the effects of such crises. These perspectives, chiefly coming from anthropology, begin to suggest that there are deeper (more hidden or latent), or implicit levels of ritual symbols along with their *on the surface* or explicit functions.

Table P.1 depicts definitions and descriptions of ritual, corresponding disciplines of authors, and citations. Their approaches to explaining ritual may assist in gaining a snapshot of the diversity of perspectives on ritual overall, including classic views.

This table only partially addresses the incredible amount of literature available on ritual. The discipline of anthropology predominates, while other disciplines have based much of their work on that of social and cultural anthropologists.

Elements, Functions, and Types of Rituals

The elements of ritual offered here come from an assorted set of texts and interpretations of writings on the subject. The amalgamation offered is intuitive and literature-based, combined to help analyze the complex topic of ritual.

Rituals operate in the context of societies with distinct cultures; they are evidence of communal bonds. They have structure, a beginning, middle, and an end (Achterberg et al., 1994), and are often described as solutions to crises and a way of dealing with and reducing the effects of crises. Ritual action is standardized, repetitive, prescribed, required, and commanded by the rules of social group, whether a culture or a subculture. The social group sets both the occasions and the forms of such ritual (Gluckman, 1975, p. 4). Rituals involve stereotypy: a certain degree of formality, rigidity, simplicity of movement, repetitiveness, and rhythm; they have a communicative function and are a response to anxiety (Davis, 1981). It is likely that the repetitiveness and prescriptive patterns of rituals and their connection to crisis situations generate much of their associated negativity.

Words, actions, objects, gestures, and relationships are important to ritual performance (Douglas, 1966; Malinowski, 1992; McCreery, 1979; Tambia, 1968; Turner, 1969; van Gennep, 1960). Symbols stand out in rituals; they are essential to ritual performance. They challenge both participants in rituals and observers of ritual to interpret meanings that are not necessarily conscious. Symbols represent condensed meaning and operate as a "cognitive reflex" (Munhall, 2007, citing Fetterman, 1989, p. 36). Because of the importance of symbols to understanding ritual, they need to be examined and framed by the cultural and social context in which they are generated and applied; the relationship of the symbol to the social order must be analyzed

TABLE P2
Nursing Literature on Nursing Ritual: Pros and Cons

Topic	Positive	Negative	Citation
Routine develops into ritual to alleviate anxiety. Observation of ritual alleviates in a general way with an individual's anxiety, avoiding clashes with other members of the group, or protects the member against the disapproval of the leader. Rituals continue even after the dangers or other reasons that brought them into being cease to exist. Many nursing rituals are associated with: cleanliness and order; time (speed and rigid schedules); communication (using professional language); talking to postpone action: fleeing from emotionally charged situations and withholding information from patients; and maintaining a professional attitude to preserve interpersonal distance with patients.		Much nursing care consists of prescribed routines that have evolved out of the need to budget time, effort, and money. Decisions about a patient's life in the hospital are often unconsciously made on the basis of rules or routines. Rituals maintain consistency and keep nurses from learning about patients and from correlating their own reactions. Professional rites not routinized rites should be achieved.	Schmahl (1964)
Some nursing routines have undefined meaning for individuals who perform them. Ritualism is behavior that has a special significance to the actor rather than orientation toward achieving organizational goals. Behavior is directed toward tasks contributing to goal achievement; behavior satisfies some psychological need of the individual, for example, compulsive cleanliness, status needs, or reduction of anxiety. Examples are (dysfunctional) routine taking of temperature, pulse, and respiration; nurses' notes (some positive functions); special report (medication errors and patient incidents) (ritualistic behavior in need of modification) and interruption and reassignment of nursing activities.	Ritualistic practice is sometimes beneficial: shift report serves to maintain group cohesion (latent function).	Ritualistic practice is sometimes inefficient and dysfunctional.	Walker (1967)
Participant observation case material on ritual procedures helps nurses defend against anxiety and are social acts generating and conveying meaning.	Nursing ritual practices have social and psychological meaning.		Chapman (1983)

(continued)

TABLE P2

Nursing Literature on Nursing Ritual: Pros and Cons (continued)

Topic	Positive	Negative	Citation
Narcotic count, medication administration, recording intake and output, oral temperatures, bathing patients, shift reports, etc.	Nursing rituals are a thinking nurse's enemy. Need to recognize the source of rituals, otherwise the nurse is on automatic pilot; patient care is improved on the basis of reason, nurses think, and do not rely on ritual.		Huttmann (1985)
Nurses need to support a more systematic approach to the delivery of nursing care.		Routine and ritual need to be relied on less.	Bowman (1986)
Rituals that should be abandoned because of research: for example, protective isolation; changing the urine bag; periurethral care; unclamping and clamping Foley catheters; soaking wounds in povidone-iodine; etc.		Many rituals fall short of what is intended and should be exposed and abandoned.	Huey (1986)
Nursing rituals coexist with science, technology, and procedure. Nursing rituals help nurses reaffirm some of the beliefs and values of nursing, such as doing good and avoiding harm. Nurses pass on subcultural knowledge by word of mouth and by demonstration. The embedded and hidden aspects of nursing ritual and of nurses' work illuminate that much of nurses' work may be largely unknown to the public.	A system of nursing rituals exists in hospital nursing, with latent and manifest levels of meaning. Examining nursing rituals illuminates the contribution of nursing to health care, despite the personal, profane, and sacred notions of some of the work.		Wolf (1986, 1988a, 1988b)
Bedtime ceremonials, repetitive performance of various activities to prepare the person for going to sleep, need to be encouraged for psychiatric patients. These behaviors can be distinguished from obsessive–compulsive rituals. Performance of these behaviors may indicate a journey back to health.	The therapeutic effects of following the patient's lead to use bedtime ceremonials may have therapeutic effects.		Geach (1987)

Source	Summary	Description
Walsh and Ford (1989)	Rituals and myths need to be exposed; they are ineffective and refuted by research findings.	Nursing fails itself and its patients because of traditional rituals and myths used in hospitals. Ritual action implies carrying out tasks without thinking it through in a problem-solving, logical way. Nursing rituals in clinical practice need to be exposed using findings from research. Examples include preoperative fasting, preoperative shaving, and postoperative dressing inspection and cleansing.
Bright (1990)	Therapeutic ritual created for a therapy session benefits families in conflict.	Family conflicts can be addressed through the creation and conduct of a therapeutic ritual during a therapeutic session.
Benton (1993)	Ritualized practice needs to be replaced by evidence.	Research-based practice needs to replace ritual in nursing.
Holland (1993)	Nursing rituals perpetuate traditional knowledge and practices and are essential for ensuring that order is maintained in a much wider social context.	Day-to-day activities are rituals and are not special. Handover report ensures that social order is maintained within the group by enforcing cohesion and interaction; reflects the values of the group. Putting on the uniform helps nurses to fulfill their role.
Mulhall (1996)	Nurses must develop a sociological and anthropological perspective to their way of thinking.	Rituals may have important social, psychological, and protective functions. In relation to the study of death, dying, and disposal of the body, the rituals of misfortune and the rituals of social transition have obvious importance. Modern death rituals, or the lack of them, in Western societies have been cited as a potential cause of the increased rate of death among the recently bereaved.
Biley and Wright (1997)	Nurses need to explore the meaning or latent function of nursing routine and ritual.	Rituals may have positive action, ritualistic symbolism latent functions, and meanings for patients and nurses beyond the instrumental function of ritual; acknowledge the value of ritual in modern health care practices.
Suominen et al. (1997)	It is important to understand the purpose and meaning of symbols and rituals, because a nursing practice goal is to provide nursing care on the basis of culture.	Culture has to do with the deep and invisible structures in society that are transferred from one generation to another. Rituals form a part of a cultural system and are usually seen as a social phenomenon.

(continued)

TABLE P.2
Nursing Literature on Nursing Ritual: Pros and Cons (continued)

Topic	Positive	Negative	Citation
Nursing rituals affect nurses' ability to act as patient advocates. Ritual action underpins most of nurses' responses to act as advocates for patients.		Nursing routines and rituals serve to distance nurses from patients, to have poor advocacy skills, and serve to overcome the anxiety associated with care of the terminally ill.	Martin (1998)
Traditional nursing culture with its task orientation, rigid hierarchical structures, and resultant staff disempowerment impede the delivery of patient-centered care. Task-focused nursing centers on the nurses' need to detach from patients. Staff need to assist patients with meals and hygiene needs, not "do" patients.		Rituals, routines, and cultures developed in nursing prevent nurses from achieving individualized, person-centered holistic nursing care.	Tonuma and Winbolt (2000)
Symbols and rituals are intimately connected as are the individuals who embody the symbols or perform the rituals. Rituals communicate values and produce desired effects. Ritual is universal phenomenon inherent to all human groups and societies. Nurses need to renew their appreciation for the transformative power of nursing rituals to embrace the holistic paradigm.	Nursing symbols and rituals are significant for the practice of professional nursing.		Catanzaro (2002)

Author		
Philpin (2002)	Vigilance is needed when thinking about nursing practice, but rituals are considered useful according to social science. While research-based practice is valued over ritualized practice, the symbolic function of ritual action is promoted. There is a lack of authority for understanding ritual within nursing literature, suggesting that groups define ritual for their own purposes and arguments.	The negative usage of ritual as unthinking, routinized action by nurses misses out on the wider symbolic meaning of the word. There is much to be gained from further elaboration of the ways in which nurses use rituals in the performance of their work; they provide a rich source of insight into the meanings attached in the accomplishment of nursing care.
Denham (2003)	There are relationships among culture, family rituals, health, and illness. Family rituals are compelling and bounded behaviors with symbolic meanings that can be clearly described and serve to organize and affirm central family ideas; serve as a unifying factor for family identity and values. Definitions of family rituals and ritual types and dimensions are provided. Families in different developmental stages may find that family rituals and routines have implications for health.	Family rituals help think about potential relationships with adherence to prescribed medical regiments, therapeutic health management, and health or illness outcomes.

and understood (Douglas, 1970). Ritual activity is comprised of a high degree of symbolic input compared to other types of human activity (Davis, 1981). Symbolic objects can be physical and nonphysical.

Ritual symbols transmit cultural ideas and meanings. Symbols are "storage bins" of information; they are "not about pragmatic techniques, but about cosmologies, values, and cultural axioms, whereby a society's deep knowledge is transmitted from one generation to another" (Turner, 1974, p. 239). By analyzing ritual symbols you may get to their implicit goal (Turner, 1967, p. 45) and meaning.

Rituals can also be examined for their functions and consequences. For example, "What are their manifest functions (objective consequences contributing to the adjustment of adaptation of the system...intended and recognized by participants in the system [Merton, 1968, p. 105]; explicit, on the surface)? What are their latent functions (...neither intended nor recognized [Merton, p. 105]; implicit, hidden)." Moreover, rituals can produce a feeling of completeness; participants in rituals have experienced "a whole act, a finished sequence, the achievement (at least for a while) of satisfaction, satiation, perhaps serenity" (Kafka, 1983, p. 31).

There are many types of rituals. For example, rituals of mourning and bereavement (Skultans, 1980) help individuals express grief over the death of a loved one. In interaction rituals (Goffman, 1967), there are rules for social encounters, during face-to-face behavior, based on established requirements whereby the kinds of practices employed maintain a specified and obligatory kind of ritual equilibrium. In addition, rituals of initiation help the new members of a society perform and demonstrate worthiness for admission to a tribe or social group (Starker, 1978), as in a hospital or a nursing unit. These rituals are similar to Bosk's (1980) conceptualization of occupational ritual, where through meetings and case conferences physicians learn what it means to be a physician. Next, the corporate culture of business performs award rituals or "Attaboys," seen as dramatizations of the company's basic cultural values (Deal & Kennedy, 1982). Therapeutic or healing rituals help people to cope and become healthy (Achterberg et al., 1994; Galambos, 2001; Lakomy, 1994), while sacramental rituals in the Catholic Church reaffirm the oneness of its members in the Church and serve as "channels of grace" (Douglas, 1982, p. 8). Individual rituals are directed to the growth of one person and can be designed to meet the needs of an individual, for example, to change the meaning of an event or behavior (Galambos, 2001).

NURSING LITERATURE ON RITUAL

Accounts of nursing ritual have attracted greater or lesser attention over many decades. Early on, Virginia Walker (1967) conducted studies on common activities of nurses engaged in direct patient care and rituals. She suggested that these rituals have special significance for the nurse and satisfy some personal need. Walker studied taking vital signs, special reports (medical errors and incident reports), and charting nurses' notes. She judged the nursing rituals she concentrated on to be of little value. On the other hand, she saw them as being anxiety reducing, admitting their potential worth.

Many others have addressed nursing rituals (Catanzaro, 2002; Holland, 1993; Suominen et al., 1997; Tonuma & Winbolt, 2000; Walsh & Ford, 1989; Wolf, 1988a) and have held differing conclusions about their value. One consideration emerges when scanning the nursing literature; the definitions used by authors vary greatly. This book uses the definition of ritual by DeCraemer et al. (1976): patterned, symbolic action that refers to the goals and values of a social group (p. 469).

Even so, selections from the literature (Table P.2) have been collected intermittently over decades using search strategies with databases, mainly nursing, or have been found accidently while pursuing other topics or shared by colleagues. They stand as representatives on the topic. Not all the rituals are nursing rituals; for example, Geach's (1987) article emphasizes the importance of nurses' support of bedtime rituals for psychiatric patients.

The texts selected from sections of articles and books in Table P.2 epitomize what is a typical array on the topic: some are scholarly, some are research, and some are largely opinion. What they reveal is that the balance of opinion seems to be positive, to value the worth of not only writing about nursing rituals, but also seeing the place of nursing rituals in the larger context of professional culture.

I

Rituals of Nursing Practice

Section I includes descriptions of nursing rituals consisting of direct care activities. The background of the ritual, related traditions, ritual initiation, artistic aspects, evolving research, and ritual symbol are explored in each part.

The interpersonal caring ritual is presented in the context of interpersonal relationships. It is viewed through the literature of nursing, including caring theories, and other disciplines. As the most important nursing ritual, it provides the stage for subsequent and simultaneous nursing care. The history of nursing's association with cleanliness and hygiene frames the examination of bathing patients as a nursing ritual in transition. Nurses' association with sacred and profane aspects of life is considered. Postmortem care, the last nursing care given to patients, is framed by end-of-life care. Similar to bathing patients, postmortem care involves nurses coming into contact with bodily products considered profane, yet with human experience that is sacred. One aspect of the medication-use process, medication administration, is explored from the perspectives of patient safety. Ritual numbers and their variations in the administration function are compared.

1

Interpersonal Caring Ritual and Interpersonal Relationships

*E*veryday nursing life is composed of multiple interactions with patients in many social and cultural contexts. Yet, when nurses begin to interact with patients, they meet strangers with a need for nursing care. In many settings, nurses begin to expand their knowledge of patients by virtue of traditional health histories, nursing histories, and nursing care plans that accumulate with electronic and paper documents detailing patients' stories. Patients' situations are further explained during change-of-shift report or handoffs, as patients are admitted to or move within the units of hospitals and long-term care agencies (Heliker & Scholler-Jaquish, 2006). Their stories continue to expand. It is nurses' own experiences with patients during everyday clinical encounters that build nursing knowledge of individuals as nurses care for and learn from patients.

Nurses typically answer the call to care by greeting patients. Their greeting begins a relationship initiated during a meeting that is characteristically reciprocal as patients in turn respond to the nurses' presence. The interaction takes shape and progresses, and nurses and patients connect. The work of caring–healing is "life giving and life receiving" (Watson, 2005, p. 3). There is a "rhythmic give and take between nurses and patients" (Finfgeld-Connett, 2008a, p. 530). The relationship that develops can be interpreted as a caring one, yet the judgment about whether it is caring or not varies according to the appraisals of both participants (Godkin & Godkin, 2004). Patients' well-being and healing are at stake. Furthermore, the proposition that the interpersonal encounters between nurses and patients can be conceptualized as interventions to achieve intentional results has attracted nurse clinicians' and researchers' interest for decades (Beeber, Canuso, & Emory, 2004). This hypothesis is attributed to Hildegard Peplau (1952) and reinforced by the assertion that when there is synergy between patient characteristics and nurse characteristics, a desired outcome is likely to occur in optimal patient outcomes (Tejero, 2011).

Whether or not interpersonal caring rituals are cocreated and enacted by nurses with patients during clinical encounters is debatable. However, the performance of interpersonal caring rituals can be investigated and interpreted. So, too, can examples of ritual action be examined during nurse–patient meetings, as can the symbols nurses use when communicating with patients. In this portrayal of ritual in nursing, interpersonal caring rituals are explored from the perspective of nurse–patient interactions or relationships. It is assumed that during the enactment of interpersonal caring rituals, both nurses and patients are connected (Ranheim, Kärner, & Berterö, 2012), practically and symbolically, if only for a short time. The meaning of the ritual resides with both participants.

NURSE–PATIENT RELATIONSHIP: OPPORTUNITY FOR CARING AND RITUAL

The role of the nurse has traditionally been viewed as a provider of direct, hands-on care; the role incorporates many other responsibilities. Nursing care often involves personal knowledge of the person, frequently carried out through bodily contact that is professionally intimate (Perry, 2002). They know patients' secrets and are entrusted with them (Fagin & Diers, 1983). They initiate direct nursing care through the activities of the nurse–patient relationship; this relationship is essential to nursing and elemental to the well-being of nurses and patients (Jarrin, 2006).

Surrounding each person to be nursed is a subjective, physical space that marks his or her individual territory. Nurses enter into this space using visual, auditory, olfactory, thermal, and tactile perceptions (Hall, 1966). Nurses intrude into a patient's territory by direct access to his or her personal space. The distance between both bodies is short. Within this distance they touch patients, ask questions about bodily functions, and start IVs. Nurses also enter intimate spaces. They see patients' nakedness and provide care in a private zone. They preserve their dignity as they perform activities that patients would "do for themselves if it were at all possible" (Swanson, 1991, p. 154). Hall (1966) maintained that the physical distances individuals try to keep from others are in accordance with cultural rules. Nurses breach these boundaries and distances every day as the nursing situation evolves. Nurses who provide direct care to patients are physically present within patients' personal space (Berman, Snyder, & McKinley, 2011). The intimate relationships developed during the caring interpersonal process are shaped by expert nursing and interpersonal sensitivity (Finfgeld-Connett, 2008b).

Much of nursing care is relational and interactive. Whether physical care predominates, or emotional, psychological, and culturally appropriate support is given, nurses function in zones that are inches to several feet from patients' bodies, even when considering proximity to computer screens and interfaces during telehealth encounters. Consequently, they gain access to patients in ways that few are privileged to (Perry, 2002), including the sacred aspects of human life, such as suffering, death, grief, birth, and role transitions.

In institutional settings, nurses perform physical care: they bathe patients, administer medications, help them get out of bed, change dressings, and at the same time carry out interpersonal caring rituals during caring moments (Watson, 1988), in meetings (Paterson & Zderad, 1976), or in the nursing situation (Boykin & Schoenhofer, 2001; Paterson & Zderad, 1976). They touch patients and lay their hands to comfort and heal. They encourage patients and offer hope. They comfort patients and relieve their pain. In health care agencies, homes, and in the community or by telephone and through computers, they teach them. It is during these relational encounters that simultaneous events unfold. Practical, technical, and symbolic actions take place. The time spent together is sacred.

As nurses enter patients' personal space, they set up an environment for healing. During such interpersonal encounters, they create human caring environments whereby they use themselves consciously and intentionally to achieve the outcome of healing (Quinn, 1992). Nurses' intentions reflect their consciousness; they themselves are healing environments and creators of sacred space (Quinn, 1992). The contributions of interpersonal encounters that are authentic and intentional can have lasting benefits for patients.

In hospitals, doors are closed or curtains are pulled around a nurse and a patient to enclose both in a private space and protect the patient from passersby. The enclosure symbolizes the privacy needed by both involved in the encounter. In homes, nurses ask family members to leave the room if this is acceptable to the patient. If care is provided telephonically or via computer, privacy is ideally maintained during the dialogue.

As nurses begin to establish an interpersonal relationship with patients, they carry out a series of activities. For actions to be seen as caring, nurses must be aware of the need for care in patients; they must know that certain things could be done to improve the situation (Gaut, 1983). Nurses must intend to do something for patients and must choose an action aimed at serving as a means for bringing about a positive change in them. Next, they must carry out that action. Ultimately, the positive change must be judged on the basis of what is good for that patient rather than for the nurse or others (Gaut, 1983). The welfare of the patient is paramount.

As caring and support are offered in nurse–patient relationships, nurses must be aware of the value of interpersonal activities, such as verbal content and/or nonverbal communication actions (e.g., gestures, facial expressions, inflections placed on words, and silences) (Beeber et al., 2004). One hospital implemented a relationship-based care model and observed nurses in action with patients as they demonstrated caring behaviors, using a checklist (present or absent behaviors). Verbal behaviors were expression of concern, explanation of a procedure prior to initiation, validation of physical and emotional status; sharing personal observation in response to a concern, providing assurance, and discussing a topic of concern to the patient other than the current health problem (Winsett & Hauck, 2011, p. 287). Nonverbal caring behaviors included sitting at the bedside, touching exclusive of a procedure, sustaining eye contact, entering a patient's room without being called, and providing physical comfort measures (Winsett & Hauck, 2011, p. 287). This interpretation of nurse caring behaviors shows that in the space created by the nurse–patient relationships, actions indicating caring are observable.

When nurses enter the personal space of patients, they may use three types of touch during an interpersonal encounter: task-oriented, caring, and protective (Fredriksson, 1999). Task-oriented touch is represented as procedural, instrumental, or working touch. Caring touch, such as nonverbal communication, is also known as positive affective touch, expressive touch, nonprocedural touch, comforting touch, or unnecessary touch. Protective touch helps nurses distance themselves from emotional pain, preserve energy resources, and release tension. In Fredriksson's model, presence, touch, and listening connect people. Hearing, task-oriented touch, and being there are also evident. Fredriksson saw nurses' caring, connective touch, intentional silence, and concentrated listening to others as symbolic gifts for patients. An invitation or call from the patient allows the nurse to come into the patient's world. Both share in the narrative of the patient's suffering (Fredriksson, 1999). Two types of connection are accomplished: high intersubjectivity (being with) and minimum intersubjectivity (being there).

Another author (Routasalo, 1999) conducted an integrative review on forms of touch represented in nursing studies. The investigator classified the types of studies on the basis of touch: uses of touch, effects of touch, and experiences of touch. Body parts touched most frequently were hands, arms, forehead, hair, and shoulders. Caring touch was associated with largely emotional contact. The researcher concluded that physical touch, especially expressive touch, was not necessarily present in all nurse–patient interactions (Routasalo, 1999).

According to Engebretson (2002), hands-on nursing may represent the fundamental human connection nurses use to help patients heal.

> The metaphor of hands-on care with the intent to heal combines the heart in compassion with the head in a conscious intent to help. The ubiquitous hand is the symbolic metaphor of embodied intent to act. Thus, hands-on has always represented the activity of nursing as more than mental understanding or compassionate caring, but it must be integrated with an action toward to patient. (p. 30)

Engebretson (2002) pointed out the use of head, heart, and hand during intentional action. The need for nurses to accomplish high technology–high touch care is framed by the core commitment of professional nursing to maintain caring with the intent to heal.

Even though communication is often challenging and difficult, considering the complex situations in which nurses and patients participate, nurses still are determined to connect with each person's core. This is particularly problematic for nurses caring for patients who are locked in, unconscious, in vegetative states, or are infants. The following description illustrates a nurse's intention to reach a patient:

> A patient...could only communicate through his eyes, there was pain, yes, and anxiety in those eyes...we had eye contact until he closed them. ...He didn't speak, but spoke...through his body...then the patient didn't feel alone, we shared. [T]hat's what I hope was a help, but I can't be entirely sure, you never can, although I try to do what I believe. (Arman, 2007, pp. 88–89)

What nurses say and do is guided by the ethical principles of human dignity, autonomy, and caritas (Clarke, Watson, & Brewer, 2009; Fredriksson & Eriksson, 2003). Nurses respect themselves and their patients; they recognize the autonomy of both nurses and patients in the nursing situation, and they are motivated by caritas or compassion, originating in human love and charity (Fredriksson & Eriksson, 2003).

The real work of nursing, as hands-on care, implies nurses' connection with patients and the intent to participate in the healing of self and others (Sharoff, 2009). It is through ordinary yet extraordinary nurse–patient interactions that relationships exist that potentially heal both. Some of these relationships represent profound moments (Sharoff, 2009) or "moments of intimate connection—the occasions in which both nurses and patient feel transformed (even if only for the day) for having made it through a challenging time together" (Swanson, 1999, p. 55).

TRADITIONS, BELIEFS, AND DEFINITIONS

Interpersonal relationships created by nurses with patients are highly valued by professional nurses. This is illustrated by the concern nurses have voiced about balancing high-tech care with interpersonal caring. The contributions of both to patient outcomes is indisputable and dramatized in the technologically intense intensive care environment (Almerud, Alapack, Fridlund, & Ekebergh, 2008). Patients and machines may be easily fused in this setting.

Nurses' attention to comforting patients can be lured away by technology and laboratory results. Nurses' caring comportment is challenged. Patients may not be given much chance to talk, and at times technology intrudes into limited opportunities to do so. Nurses may fear that dialogues with patients may evoke questions and emotions not easily handled. Rather than making space for social, emotional, physical, and spiritual support, they may "pick sides" and defer to technology (Almerud et al., 2008, p. 136). In spite of technology becoming a priority for nurses in intensive care environments, nurses intend to be with patients and maintain relationships with them through compassion (Kongsuwan & Locsin, 2011).

Morse, Solberg, Neander, Bottorff, and Johnson (1991) examined conceptualizations of caring, adequacies and inadequacies of the conceptualizations, applicability of caring as concepts to the nursing profession, and trends and gaps in caring research. Five categories of caring reported were: caring as a human trait (human mode of being), caring as a moral imperative or ideal fundamental value (preserve human dignity), caring as an affect (emotional involvement with empathetic feeling for patient experience), caring as an interpersonal relationship (interaction between nurse and patient expresses and defines caring), and caring as a therapeutic intervention (caring actions such as attentive listening, patient teaching, patient advocacy, touch, being there, technical competence). Outcomes of caring identified included caring as the subjective experience of the patient and caring as a physical response. Morse et al.'s (1991) analysis provided a model and definitions for future studies of nurse caring. Not only do elements of the model validate Peplau's (1952) views, but interpersonal relationship emerge as a construct important to the study of caring.

INTERACTION RITUAL AND INTERPERSONAL CARING RITUAL

Goffman (1967), a sociologist, analyzed ritual elements in social interaction. He noted that when people interact face-to-face, the behaviors exhibited include glances, gestures, positioning, and verbal statements (Goffman, 1967). During social encounters involving face-to-face or mediated contact, individuals act out a line or a pattern of verbal and nonverbal acts by which they express their view of the situation, and their evaluation of the participants, especially themselves.

The face is the positive social value a person effectively claims for himself or herself by the line others assume he or she has taken during a particular contact. Face is a self-delineated image of approved social attributes and an image that others may share, "as when a person makes a good showing for his profession or religion by making a good showing for himself" (Goffman, 1967, p. 5).

According to Goffman, rituals are present in everyday interactions and all interactions attempt to maintain the sacredness of the group. Applying this formulation to interpersonal relationships in nursing, the social interactions created by nurses and patients during nursing situations are ritual ceremonies whereby participants value the group, the nursing profession, and the social self, the nurse and the patient, as an object of sacred reverence. Goffman's work helps make a case for interpersonal caring ritual in nursing by emphasizing ritual in social interaction and the sacredness of social interactions.

CARING THEORIES AS FRAMEWORK FOR CARING RITUAL

Interpersonal caring rituals can be framed from the perspective of nursing theories on caring and a caring science orientation. This model of science enables nurses to study the sacred in caring–healing work (Watson, 2005, p. xi). Those intent on understanding caring science aim to focus on developing a "deeper perspective on life and caring–healing work" (Watson, 1999, p. xii). Perhaps in striving to explore and understand caring science, nurses and others will "allow science, morality, metaphysics, art, and spirituality to co-mingle for new reasons" (Watson, 2005, p. xiii). Aspects of the intersubjective nature of the nurse–patient relationship and interpersonal caring rituals are clarified by selected caring theories.

Humanistic Nursing: Josephine Paterson and Loretta Zderad

Paterson and Zderad suggested that nursing implies a special kind of meeting of human persons; nurses have a goal and patients may have one too. Nurses are goal-directed toward nurturing patients and their well-being (Paterson & Zderad, 1976).

Nursing involves a mode of being and doing something (Paterson & Zderad, 1976, p. 13). Framed by a phenomenologic view of nursing in the lived world, the theorists positioned Humanistic Nursing Theory as a living out of nurses' authentic commitment and existential involvement with patients. Nurses are present "with the whole of…being" (p. 15) in personal and professional ways. Their involvement is based on art and science.

Paterson and Zderad proposed that nurses and patients relate to one another intersubjectively, or subject to subject. They also relate subject to object. Both are unique and come together with past and current social relationships. When nurses relate to patients and are present to them, they are open and receptive, ready and available to interact in a reciprocal manner. Nurses are "open-as-a-helper to the patient" (1976, p. 25). Nurses and patients relate in dialogue through call and response (George, 2002) addressing health needs (Parker, 1993).

According to Paterson and Zderad, nursing is a lived dialogue. As an intersubjective transaction, nurses and patients make choices. In the case of patients unable to choose, nurses support patients' points of view most likely solicited from family and friends and obtained from health care documents. Furthermore, each nursing event with patients is a unique, one-of-a-kind intersubjective transaction.

In Humanistic Nursing Theory, the nursing situation is created as nurses meet patients. It is focused on "lived time and space as experienced by the patient and/or nurse, and as shared intersubjectively" (Paterson & Zderad, 1976, p. 19). Interpersonal caring ritual can be explained through selected formulations of this theory. The ritual takes place in the nursing situation during meetings of nurses and patients, which are shared events. As a socially and existentially constructed space, it is often very private, very reciprocal, and very dependent on what both bring to the occasion. The ritual action, however, is demonstrated by intentional nursing where some nursing wisdom resides. Nursing wisdom builds through experience as nurses bring past experience to present nursing situations.

Caring Theory: Jean Watson

Watson's Caring Theory has garnered worldwide attention, no doubt because of its emphasis on caring, ethics, and consciousness, and on nurses and patients in a transpersonal relationship. It answers the hunger for human connection of the nurses who provide care and the patients who receive it. The theory is based on a moral/ethical/philosophical base of love and values (Watson Caring Science Institute, 2010). As a "unitary field of consciousness and energy that transcends time, space, and physicality (unity of mind/body/spirit/nature/universe)" (Watson, 1999, p. 2), nurses as providers of health care services are honored and, in turn, honor patients or clients in the transpersonal caring relationship. Human caring and relationship-centered caring are "a foundational ethic for healing practices" (Watson, 2006, p. 51).

For Watson (1999), the transpersonal caring relationship is a special kind of human care relationship. Nurses go beyond themselves. They are well-intentioned and authentic, and convey concern about the inner life world and subjective meaning of another person who is fully embodied (Watson, n.d.). Nurses reach to deeper connections, to the spirit and the universe. The goal of the transpersonal caring relationship is to protect, enhance, and preserve dignity, humanity, wholeness, and inner harmony (Watson, 2001). Nurses' caring consciousness preserves and honors patients' embodied spirit and connection to them. The transpersonal caring relationship, as a spirit-to-spirit connection, has the potential to comfort and heal. Nurses' intentionality and consciousness transcend the physical (Watson, 2002). According to Watson, both nurses and patients are unique and connect in a mutual search for meaning and wholeness. Suffering may be transcended through the caring relationship (Watson, 2001).

The caring occasion or caring moment (i.e., focal point in space and time) (Watson, 1988/1999) occurs when nurses and patients come together in an occasion for human caring. Both have unique phenomenal fields that include the totality of human experience of feelings, bodily sensations, thoughts, spiritual beliefs, goals, expectations, environmental considerations, and meanings of perceptions. All are based on life history, present moment, and imagined future. Nurses as caregivers need to be aware of their own consciousness and authentic presence of being in caring moments with patients (Watson, 1999).

As nurses experience a transpersonal caring relationship during caring moments, nurses and patients are influenced by one another through choices and actions taking place (see Ergott, 2008). The caring occasion becomes "transpersonal" when "it allows for the presence of the spirit of both—then the event of the moment expands the limits of openness and has the ability to expand human capabilities" (Watson, 1999, pp. 116–117). The caring moment becomes part of the nurse's and patient's life history. The caring moment is a phenomenal field created by, and which is greater than, the nurse and patient, each of whom has an individual field. The moment transcends the here and now. Healing occurs when the nurse connects with the spirit of the patient (Watson, 2006).

Watson's formulations of the transpersonal caring relationship and caring moment provide a space and time for nurses and patients to heal. Within this phenomenal field, caring is communicated through nurses' "energetic patterns of consciousness, intentionality, and authentic presence in caring relationship" (Watson, 2005, p. 7).

Nursing as Caring: Anne Boykin and Savina Schoenhofer

Boykin and Schoenhofer's (2001) Theory of Nursing as Caring assumes that all persons are caring and that caring is an essential characteristic of being human. Humans' wholeness is celebrated in their theory. Nurses offer caring in the context of the caring situation that is a shared, lived experience in which caring between the nurse and the nursed enhances personhood. Personhood is the process of living grounded in caring and enhanced through nurturing relationships. Nurses and patients are together valued and respected and energized in the caring situation. Nursing's focus is in nurturing persons, living caring, and growing in caring (Boykin & Schoenhofer, 2001).

Consistent with the Theory of Nursing as Caring, nurses and patients are whole persons; nurses' awareness of themselves as caring persons includes their consciousness to value caring and leads to the question: "How ought I act as caring person?" (Boykin & Schoenhofer, 2001, p. 4). Caring relationships express the fullness of being human and living caring each day. "A relationship experienced through caring holds at its heart the importance of person-as-person" (p. 4). An ongoing, authentic awareness of self is necessary to developing caring relationships, knowing self, and knowing others. Nurses as caring persons live caring and have the potential to participate in nurturing relationships by caring for others. Boykin and Schoenhofer contended that the profession of nursing applies knowledge gained from investigations conducted by the discipline and in response to human needs.

Theory of Caring and Uncaring: Sigridur Halldorsdottir

Sigridur Halldorsdottir (1996) proposed a Theory of Caring and Uncaring Behaviors that she developed from phenomenologic studies. She connected caring to patient outcomes and pointed out the potential of nurse–patient relationships for helping patients heal. Halldorsdottir emphasized the value of each human, the importance of relationships, the interdependence of humans, and the source of human suffering to be comprised of unmet needs.

Halldorsdottir described five basic approaches to being with another, presented as a continuum, to represent caring interactions. The biogenic mode of being is the approach where nurses or other health care providers as professionals recognize the personhood of clients through caring interactions. They strengthen clients, promote their healing, and reduce their vulnerability. Patients feel a sense of well-being. The bioactive mode is life-sustaining, and nurses and other providers support, encourage, and reassure clients. Clients are comforted. The biopassive or life-neutral mode of being occurs when clients perceive neither positive nor negative influences on their well-being. Next, the biostatic mode of being is life-restraining; providers are seen as indifferent or insensitive to clients' needs. The biocidic mode of being results in clients feeling depersonalized and vulnerable. This mode is most destructive for clients. All of these modes of being take place during nurse–client encounters.

During nurse–client encounters, nurses openly communicate and connect with patients. They demonstrate compassion and respect. The potential for uncaring is also there; in this case, nursing and other providers are disconnected, indifferent, and incompetent. Clients are discouraged (Halldorsdottir, 1996, 2007).

These caring theories reinforce the importance of nurse–patient relationships for professional nursing. Together, the caring moment, occasion, meeting, or situation provide the space and time for the development of the relationship. Values, such as respect and dignity, converge and the wholeness of nurses and patients are emphasized. Both nurse and patient benefit as they interact and grow.

RELATIONSHIP AND RITUAL

When nurses approach patients and begin a nurse–patient relationship, they participate compassionately in the experience. They are aware of the "pain and brokenness of the other" (Roach, 2002, p. 50). Nurses are responsible for alleviating suffering (Morse, Bottorff, Anderson, O'Brien, & Solberg, 1992). Helping patients is their mission (Perry, 2002). The weight of the relationship is carried by nurses; they intend to care for patients, to lessen their suffering, and to heal them. The quality of nurses' presence in the encounter allows them to share with patients and make room for them (Roach, 2002). However, compassion or caritas is not always visible behaviorally.

Much of what transpires between nurses and patients comes about interpersonally, interactively, and transpersonally and is implicit or hidden to outside observers. This is not surprising because what nurses bring to the caring situation is shaped by beliefs and culture as it is reciprocally shaped by the beliefs and cultures of patients and family members in the situation. What follows is a variety of visible behaviors and verbal and nonverbal exchanges. Some patients are not responsive to nurses verbally or nonverbally. It is then up to nurses to gauge their effectiveness and to analyze whether the interactions were caring.

Nurses' personalities, actions, and expertise as well as patients' circumstances shape the nursing situation in the relational encounter. Often, what nurses learn about how to carry out interpersonal relationships is developed by trial and error and by assimilating the techniques of mentor nurses. Performance is gradually enhanced by experience and reflection on experience as maturation and insights develop (Finfgeld-Connett, 2008a).

Within the nurse–patient relationship, as nurses engage with patients who suffer, responses are triggered and nurses identify with patients' experiences through empathetic insight. They attend to the objectiveness and abstract the conditions of patients as patients remain at the center

(Morse et al., 1992). Nurses may use more energy as they engage with suffering patients to reduce suffering, rather than merely responding by rote. However, pseudoinvolvement, described as being detached and disembodied or disengaged, could take place, resulting in a nontherapeutic nurse–patient interaction. This outcome is always a possibility in nurse–patient relationships.

Interpersonal caring rituals take place at an individual level between the nurse and the patient and also function at a social level in the context of professional nursing. The interpersonal caring ritual provides meaning for nurses and patients and establishes order for their interactions and mutual experiences. The meaning of the relationship as experienced is realized through reflecting on experience. Nurses must make sense of the nurse–patient relationship in the context of the caring situation or moment and in the wider context of professional nursing.

Interpersonal caring rituals evidence both common and individualized activities displayed by nurses within the boundary of the nurse–patient relationship. In the relational encounters of nurses and patients, the words spoken, gestures used, and positions of nurses' bodies evidence ritual activity. The ritual performance is often private, not witnessed by others, yet represents the nurse's personal values as well as the core values of professional nursing. The nursing encounter or situation provides the space and time for nurse–patient relationships and interpersonal caring rituals.

INITIATION TO INTERPERSONAL RELATIONSHIPS

The ability to establish and sustain interpersonal relationships is a core competency for nurses (Christiansen, 2009). So when nursing students begin clinical placements in health care agencies, they often begin to communicate with patients before demonstrating other nursing skills. Although many nursing programs do not screen applicants for the ability to be compassionate and hold values consistent with those of professional nursing practices, faculty expect nursing students to be caring and respect human dignity.

Many nursing programs have incorporated reflective practice methods into nursing student assignments. Faculty believe that reflective practice helps students to make sense of events, situations, and actions that occur in clinical agencies. They encourage students to evaluate their impact on meeting patients' needs and to determine their personal growth as beginning nurses.

Therapeutic communication is emphasized in nursing education programs using nursing fundamentals textbooks in support of student learning. It receives greater attention when students take psychiatric–mental health nursing courses (Antai-Otong, 2008; Gilje, Klose, & Birger, 2007) when therapy shifts the focus to more specific interventions. The imperative to be therapeutic challenges faculty and students alike, particularly when considering the efforts of students to communicate with patients during first clinical encounters. The classic model of sender, message, receiver, and feedback-response is often presented and verbal communication models are explained with examples (Berman et al., 2011). Recently, students have begun to learn and practice SBAR (Situation, Background, Assessment, and Recommendation) to improve communication to health care providers and reduce errors (Manning, 2006). In addition, therapeutic communication, used in a helping and goal-directed relationship, may be characterized as demonstrating attentive listening and physical attending. Attentive listening focuses on patients' needs and communicates caring and interest to encourage their response. Physical attending includes listening, being present or with the patient, using posture to communicate openness, and maintaining eye contact (Berman et al., 2011).

Techniques of therapeutic communication are listed in fundamentals of nursing textbooks, such as using silence, providing general leads, being specific and tentative, using open-ended questions, using touch, restating or paraphrasing, seeking clarification, and perception checking or seeking consensual validation. Additional techniques are: offering self, giving information, acknowledging, clarifying time or sequence, presenting reality, focusing, reflecting, and summarizing and planning (Berman et al., 2011, pp. 310–311). Phases of the helping relationship are taught: preinteraction phase, introductory phase, working phase, and termination phase (Berman et al., 2011). Later in the curriculum, phases of the nurse–patient or client relationship are reviewed as well, including orientation, identification, exploitation, and resolution (Antai-Otong, 2008). Active listening, identification with patients' feelings, putting one's self in patients' shoes, being honest, genuine, credible, and ingenious or creative, being aware of cultural differences, maintaining confidentiality, and knowing role and limitations are outlined as ways of helping patients (Berman et al., 2011).

Faculty encourage students to develop self-awareness from one patient encounter to another so that strengths and limitations are analyzed and competency develops. Faculty may require students to perform process recordings of interpersonal communication episodes (Antai-Otong, 2008). They emphasize the development of a rapport with patients and supervise students' growth via this assignment.

Students develop skills in the nurse–patient relationship gradually. They learn to interact and hopefully reflect on experiences with patients as they progress in undergraduate nursing curriculums. However, the development of self-awareness is not easy, particularly when students do not practice reflection or introspection. One investigator (Scheick, 2011) made a case for students to practice mindfulness. She pointed out that students bring their own unfinished conflicts to relationships with patients. Mindful aliveness then helps students to be fully attentive to patients as persons; students invest themselves consciously in the present nurse–client moment. Self-control involves students being resolute and taking charge about choices in their lives, and self-concept behavior means that students are self-aware, open to themselves, and conscious of paying attention to inner thoughts and emotions. Although the sample size was small for experimental and control groups, some trends were promising regarding attentiveness in experimental group results.

Nursing's oral tradition is strong in relation to the transmission of cultural knowledge. Because of this, expert clinicians participate by example in mentoring neophytes. It is likely that the skilled activities nurses use when creating interpersonal relationships with patients pass on to observers and are incorporated into their personal repertory of interactive strategies.

ARTISTIC INTERPERSONAL RELATIONSHIPS

Artistic interpersonal relationships are fundamental to expert nursing practice. Consistent with this belief is the argument posed by Johnson (1994). She described nursing art as "the nurse's ability to grasp meaning in patient encounters, the nurse's ability to establish a meaningful connection with the patient, the nurse's ability to skillfully perform nursing activities, the nurse's ability to rationally determine an appropriate course of nursing action, and the nurse's ability to morally conduct his or her nursing practice" (p. 3). Grasping meaning in patient encounters is accomplished by nurses who understand what is significant in a particular patient situation. Establishing a meaningful connection with patients refers to an attachment or union between nurses and patients that promotes authenticity, wholeness, and integrity in the encounter and engagement that involves subject-to-subject interaction. Next, skillfully performing nursing activities requires demonstrating proficiency and dexterity in meeting patients' needs while performing tasks, procedures, and techniques. Rationally determining an appropriate course of nursing action suggests that the intellectual abilities of nurses lead them to draw conclusions based on knowledge, including science, and the ability to arrive at the best possible outcome for patients. Lastly, nurses are motivated by moral values framing their care and concern for patients (Johnson, 1994, pp. 4–12). Johnson's argument reinforces the essential nature and elements of the nurse–patient relationship for nursing practice and hints at how artistic performances by expert nurses accompany other nursing functions. "[In nursing as in art] you're trying to creatively intervene with a patient and help them heal...it's very abstract..." (Skillman-Hull, 1994, p. 119).

Benner (2000) also considered artistic nursing performance. She represented caring clinical practices as actions based on knowledge and a commitment to meet patients and families in their life worlds. She valued the insights gained from stories of clinical practice, noting that caring practices are revealed in such accounts. Benner emphasized that artful caring practices are knowledgeable, lifesaving, and not perfect. Expert performances are revealed in this way:

> *...we know them when we experience them, and we recognize them when they are missing. Nothing less than safe passage through diagnosis and therapy, with a sense of integrity and dignity, is at stake when excellent nursing practice is eroded.* (Benner, 2000)

Another discussion of nursing art positioned it in Eriksson's theory (Nåden & Eriksson, 2000, citing Eriksson), whereby the ultimate essence of caring is the alleviation of patients' suffering and the fundamental motivation is charitable. Framed by this theory, nurses invite patients into interaction as they turn toward them (Nåden & Eriksson, 2000) literally and figuratively at the starting point of nurse–patient relationships. Acceptance of patients begins with nurses recognizing them; acceptance serves as a foundation for the relationship. Similarly, the relationship is based on nurses confirming patients, that is, their attitudes are inviting and their behavior is calm. Patients' experiences, existence, and their right to feel what they feel are respected. By communicating invitation and confirmation, patients are brought forward into the relationship. The expressions on patients' faces, through their gazes, appeal to nurses. The nurse is ethically responsible to answer this call. Developing expertise at invitation and confirmation epitomize nursing art in interpersonal relationships.

RESEARCH ON CARING RELATIONSHIPS

Table 1.1 presents a selection of citations representing the evolution of research on interpersonal relationships in nursing and caring relationships over 10 years. A variety of research designs were used in the studies. Both patients' and nurses' perspectives were elicited.

INTERPERSONAL CARING RITUAL AND SYMBOLS

An interpersonal caring ritual is therapeutic in that it aims to improve the welfare, well-being, and condition of patients. It can heal patients and nurses. The ritual performance reaffirms the personal and professional values and beliefs of nurses. It enacts nurses' respect for the dignity of all persons and nurses' interest in doing good work. Nurses are compassionate as they commit to decreasing patients' suffering, answer patients' calls for nursing, and respond to the needs of patients. As an enactment of caring, it expresses human love and charity (Råholm & Lindholm, 1999).

TABLE 1.1
Reviewed Citations

Study/ Article	Theoretical Basis for Study	Design; Question/Purpose; Sampling Frame/Size	Independent Variables (IV); Dependent Variables (DV)	Measurement of Variables (Name of Instrument, etc.)	Statistics Used to Answer Research Question	Findings
Fredriksson (1999)	Caring relationship is the basis of caring (Paterson & Zderad, 1998); caring motive is to alleviate suffering (Eriksson, 1992)	Qualitative research synthesis; to develop an ontologic and theoretical understanding of presence, touch, and listening in a caring conversation; to describe and develop a deeper understanding of each concept by means of research synthesis of qualitative caring and nursing studies; to describe tentatively the relations between the concepts; 28 studies with 262 informants	Caring conversation, research synthesis on presence, touch, and listening	Hermeneutic circle		Two modes of relating in a caring conversation: connection with high intersubjectivity and contact with limited intersubjectivity

Caring presence: being there (physical presence, communication, understanding); being with (interpersonal and intersubjective mode of being; gift and invitation to make room for the other person; patient invites nurse to see, share, touch, and hear the brokenness, vulnerability, and suffering)

Touch, contact and noncontact types (task-oriented touch as procedural, instrumental, or working touch; caring touch as nonverbal communication, also known as positive affective touch, expressive touch, nonprocedural touch, comforting touch, or non-necessary touch; protective touch helps nurses distance themselves from emotional pain, preserve energy resources, and release tension); touch a form of relating

Listening: as an intentional act; taking in all aspects of patients' message; allowing them time and space to think and tell the story; process; deliberate and active behavior; paying attention to the speaker; demands conscious effort, searches for meaning and understanding, creative activity essential to establish relationship |

Villanueva (1999)	Conceptual orientation: patient recollections of experiences during coma or after sedation; communication behaviors of critical care nurses	Qualitative, grounded theory; to explore the experience of critical care nurses caring for unresponsive neuroscience ICU patients (in traumatic coma or pharmacologic paralysis): what type of care did the nurse provide to these patients? When did the nurse talk to the patient? What did the nurse talk about to the patient? What factors promoted or inhibited talking to the patient? How did the nurse assess the patient's comfort needs? What interventions did the nurse perform to provide patient comfort? What do nurses believe a patient perceives while receiving NMBAs? 16 critical care nurses	Experiences of critical care nurses caring for unresponsive patients	Interviews, grounded theory method	Core category: Giving the patient a chance; subcategories: Learning about the patient (gathering information; isolating subtle changes; interpreting needs); maintaining and monitoring (focusing on the technical); watching out for the patient (looking for change, keeping the patient safe, getting the patient comfortable, maintaining a delicate balance, making clinical judgments); talking to my patient (instructing the patient, reassuring the patient, providing individualized conversation); working with families (establishing a relationship, teaching the family, motivating the family, protecting the family, working around the family); struggling with dilemmas (forgetting there is a person, judging the patient); personalizing the experience (wanting to be talked to, needing family and friends, being medicated, having privacy, listening to the radio or television, having some quiet time) Many factors influence talking to the patient (characteristics of individual nurse, condition of patient, patient-related information, circumstances of injury, families, length of staff employment in unit) Doing everything to help the patient attain the best possible outcome
Carroll, 2004	Importance of quality communication to quality nursing practice;	Metasynthesis; what characterizes nonvocal ventilated patients' perceptions of being understood across qualitative studies;	Metaphors translated study to study:	Analysis: Paterson (2001); Thorne & Paterson (1998)	Overarching themes: Characteristics of communication : Not Being Understood: inequality of communication, misunderstandings, altered perceptions; loss of control: unmet needs, dependency, dehumanization; negative emotions

(continued)

TABLE 1.1

Reviewed Citations (continued)

Study/ Article	Theoretical Basis for Study	Design; Question/Purpose; Sampling Frame/Size	Independent Variables (IV); Dependent Variables (DV)	Measurement of Variables (Name of Instrument, etc.)	Statistics Used to Answer Research Question	Findings
	Peplau's interpersonal relations theory (1992)	to provide an enlarged interpretation and understanding and to build cumulative knowledge of the communication experiences of the nonvocal ventilated patients' perceptions of being understood; 12 studies; 111 participants	communication experience of nonvocal ventilated patients			Nursing care desired: individualized care, caring presence. Nurses have a critical role in facilitating communication in nonvocal ventilated patients.
Johansson, Skärsäter, and Danielson (2007)	Encounter as a prerequisite for building relationship, cornerstone of psychiatric nursing; encounters in psychiatric and mental health settings; basic understanding of what it means to be human	Qualitative, focused ethnography; to describe encounters in health care environment on locked psychiatric ward (acutely ill patients with affective and eating disorders)	Encounters on locked psychiatric ward	Participant observation of encounters in dining and day room and patients' activity room, smoking room, corridor rooms, informal interviews, document analysis, field notes; analysis (Krippendorff, 2004)		Caring relationship: personal relationships: between staff and patients, staff and next of kin, between patients, patients and next of kin and friends; staff treated patients with respect and ensured that staff-patient interactions from previous stays on ward were well established; staff took advantage of various opportunities; physical and spiritual closeness between staff members and patients Uncaring relationship: failure to create or maintain a caring relationship; failed to show respect by not adhering to rules of confidentiality, not taking patient seriously, being too personal; staff distant resulting in difficulties with establishing contact; lack of trust on part of patients and staff

Author (year)					Findings
	was the common ground for being in the world with patients				Unrecognized relationship: patient relationships with each other; patients involved in each other's care Encounters led to personal relationships characterized by caring and uncaring relationships
Finfgeld-Connett (2007)	Importance of caring in nursing; caring, the essence of nursing; lack of clarity on caring	Metasynthesis; to enhance understanding of concept of caring; how can caring be better understood by using an inductive metasynthesis approach; 6 qualitative report; 49 concept analyses	Process of caring	Grounded Theory method (Strauss & Corbin, 1998)	Caring is an interpersonal process, characterized by expert nursing, interpersonal sensitivity, and intimate relationships Antecedent to caring process: physical, psychosocial, and/or spiritual needs for andopenness to caring on part of care recipient Antecedent care provider preconditions: professional maturity, moral underpinnings, and conducive work environment Consequences: patients' physical and mental well-being; nurses' mental well-being
Finfgeld-Connett (2008a)	Presence, caring, and art of nursing in previous studies	Theory development; to examine and integrate similarities among the art of nursing, presence, and caring via inductive process	Theoretical framework development of nursing practice based on qualitative investigations on art of nursing, presence, and caring	Aggregation of qualitative findings (studies and metasyntheses) related to the art of nursing, presence, and caring	Theoretical framework of nursing practice: involves the context of a conducive environment whereby the patient perceives a need for and is open to a therapeutic relationship with the nurse; a relationship-centered intimate partnership develops: the nurse uses and creatively adapts personal and professional knowledge on the basis of values; nursing interventions are situation-specific, holistic, and accomplish patient empowerment; the patient outcome is enhanced with physical and psychological well-being; the nurse outcome is enhanced with psychological well-being Nurse–patient interaction is relationship-centered, characterized by rhythmic give-and-take between nurse and patient. The cyclic interpersonal process is characterized by authenticity and trust

(continued)

TABLE 1.1
Reviewed Citations (continued)

Study/ Article	Theoretical Basis for Study	Design; Question/Purpose; Sampling Frame/Size	Independent Variables (IV); Dependent Variables (DV)	Measurement of Variables (Name of Instrument, etc.)	Statistics Used to Answer Research Question	Findings
Brown (2009)	Stress in workplace, self-care in work environment	Qualitative, phenomenologic; to assess the meaning of caring for self by registered nurse leaders who participated in holistic caring-for-self project; 10 nurse leaders managers in acute-care hospital, purposive sample		Interviews with additional follow-up, open-ended questions; hermeneutic phenomenology (van Manen, 1990)		Metaphor: climbing to the mountain peak as journey of life; upward climb metaphor for care of self and challenge to incorporate care of self in their lives Reflection on the journey; why to care for self on the journey; how to care for self on the journey; wisdom learned along the path
Henricson, Segesten, Berglund, and Määtä (2009)	Conceptual orientation on touch; tactile touch uses effleurage used to touch the skin using slow strokes with firm pressure, mainly performed by trained touch therapists with flat of hand with fingers close together	Qualitative, phenomenologic; to illuminate the meaning of receiving tactile touch when being cared for in an intensive care unit; six former ICU patients following discharge	Tactile touch	Interviews using broad and open questions and follow-up questions; analysis methods of Ricoeur (1992), Lindseth and Norberg (2004)		Imagined room of togetherness comprising patient and touch therapist; private area with opportunity to focus on oneself. Receiving tactile touch gives hope to patients during intensive care Main theme: Being connected to oneself—enjoying comfort (one's body, mind, and memories); being connected to time (enjoy slowness, longing for continuity, being in reality): Being in togetherness (being in privacy, being in reciprocal trust, being privileged, focusing on oneself) Main theme: Being unable to gain and maintain pleasure—being exposes to annoying stimuli (being exposed to unpleasant feelings, being moved to another surrounding);

Citation	Theoretical concept	Design and purpose	Concept studied	Data source and analysis	Findings
Christiansen (2009)	Students' development of authentic concern as they communicate with patients; Martinsen (1997, 2000), Jourard (1971), Goffman (1959)	Qualitative, microethnography, longitudinal; to examine the ways students shape their role as nurses: how do students express authentic concern in relationships with patients; four second-year nursing students, during second and third years of program	Authentic concern development in relationship	Videotapes of four students assisting patients with morning care (four episodes each), semistructured interviews; analysis (Alvesson & Sköldberg, 1994; Hammersley & Atkinson, 1987)	being exposed to an annoying environment (being interrupted by the staff and the surroundings); being left without comforting touch (being abandoned; being one among many again) Students expressed their attitude toward patient through body movement, voice, and type They differed from each other: they moved easily or were less spontaneous; the body was used as a tool adapted to the situation; situation-based humor was used Students must develop their personal style in correlation with expectations of nurse's role and commit to and become involved in patients' experiences Students need to work on their own expression to maintain important norms in developing patient relationships and faculty need to be their resources
Sieger, Fritz, and Them (2011)	Interaction between nurses and patients; Paterson and Zderad (1976); Bourdieu (1977, 1990, 1992) theory of social practice and habitus	Qualitative; to investigate the situational and interactive level of action in an inpatient setting; questions: which topics are of concern to paraplegic patients after the paralysis has set in and how do nurses perceive and interpret the patient's situation;	Interactive level of action; communicative expressions of nurses and patients	Interviews, participant observation; analysis (Mayring, 1997)	Characteristics in interaction: 1. There were no negotiation processes: patient needs perceived and addressed by nurse as long as they are not in conflict with existing nursing and rehabilitation concepts 2. Patient and nurse able to negotiate: nurses and patient admit to uncertainty; nurse's approach maintains contact with patient, submits suggestions, listens to patient's point of view and adapts to patient's individual pace and integration process

(continued)

TABLE 1.1
Reviewed Citations (continued)

Study/ Article	Theoretical Basis for Study	Design; Question/Purpose; Sampling Frame/Size	Independent Variables (IV); Dependent Variables (DV)	Measurement of Variables (Name of Instrument, etc.)	Statistics Used to Answer Research Question	Findings
		how is the nursing offer negotiated with the patient and which components are decisive for the interaction process; which type of behavior of the nurses can help patients cope with their situation and be able to integrate the incident in their lives; 26 cases and 155 inquiries; 26 patients; 26 nurses				3. Patient shapes and leads: high nurse turnover rate is context; patient assumes role as case manager, compensates lack of information and arranges well-proven procedures in nursing approach upheld; tensions arise
Tejero (2011)	Synergy Model of American Association of Critical Care Nurses; dyadic relationship between nurse and patient related to patient satisfaction; mediated model	Correlational path analytic design; to test the direct and indirect relations of nurse characteristics and patient characteristics to patient satisfaction, as mediated by nurse–patient dyadic bonding; 210 nurse–patient dyads	Nurse characteristics, nurse–patient dyadic bonding, patient satisfaction	Unobtrusive observations, interviews, NPBI, observation checklist, measured nurse–patient dyadic bonding (mediating variable)	Path analysis: nurse–patient bonding (equated with bonding factor score) patient satisfaction highest coefficient (0.327), $r = 0.70$, $p = .001$	Nurse–patient dyad bonding mediates the effect of patient predictability and nurse facilitation of learning on patient satisfaction; patient predictability has direct effect on patient satisfaction; nurse facilitation of learning had indirect effect. Nurses should improve health teaching competence

NPBI, nurse–patient bonding instrument.

The interpersonal caring ritual is carried out within the boundaries of the nursing situation, occasion, moment, or meeting. The nurse–patient relationship that develops as a consequence of the encounter is foundational to clinical nursing practice. The nurse enters the patient's intimate or personal space and invites the patient's response. His or her gaze is on the patient, in most cases, eye to eye. Visual, auditory, olfactory, thermal, and tactile perceptions are integrated. While the nurse may use caring touch, other types of touch may be used if accepted by the patient. Other gestures may be evident as words are spoken and nonverbal communication techniques are used; the nurse's bodily position symbolizes both the intent to care and attentiveness. The words that the nurse uses begins with a greeting and progresses to a focus on what the nurse perceives to be the call for care. The encounter symbolizes hands-on care, even though physical contact may not be executed.

SUMMARY

Interpersonal caring rituals carried out by nurses every day are in fact dramatic, connecting encounters for nurses and patients. The importance of this ritual is confirmed by its emphasis on basic nursing programs and on nurses' preoccupation with establishing and maintaining relationships with patients. As a stage or basis of subsequent and simultaneous nursing activities it is perhaps the most important ritual of all.

2

Bathing Patients: Nursing Ritual in Transition

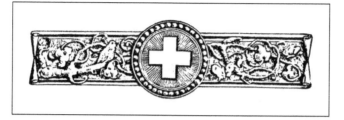

The bath, or bathing patients, has traditionally operationalized nurses' commitment to hygienic practices, cleanliness, and comfort for patients. The bath symbolizes the washing away of disease and suffering and is caring, healing work (Wolf, 1986a). As bodywork, bathing patients is at the heart of nursing (Twigg, 2002) and is rooted in the beliefs, art, and science of the profession (Wolf, 1993).

Textbooks on fundamentals of nursing provide details on how to bathe patients who are unable to perform this self-care activity for themselves. Videos are also available; they have been produced as part of a media series and are available on YouTube (Hawknurse, 2008). Nursing students learn the procedure in the beginning courses of their education programs, often through simulated experiences in nursing laboratories, and shortly thereafter with patients. At the same time, nursing students hear from RNs working in hospitals that bathing patients is not part of their jobs, that this procedure is delegated to patient care associates. Nursing assistants (NAs) also provide most of the functional care, including bathing and other bodywork activities, for residents of nursing homes (Hartig, 1998; Jervis, 2001; Rader et al., 2006; Wagnild & Manning, 1985). Some question the virtue of this delegation (Touhy, 1997).

Performance of basic care activities has declined in some instances in health care agencies (Thomson, 2009). Recent patient complaints about the absence of baths and reduced personal cleanliness in hospitals have caught nurses' attention. Nurses and family members are incredulous that they or their loved ones are not offered the opportunity to bathe or actually do not bathe while hospitalized. Consequently, patients want to leave the hospital against medical advice because they feel "grungy." At one national meeting in the United Kingdom, media attention concerning a discussion about nursing care delegated to NAs asked if nurses were "'too clever to care' and 'too posh to wash?'" (Scott, 2004). No doubt shortened hospital stays have contributed to this change. In addition, nurses found that work pressures of reduced staff, heavy workload, and the demand for efficiency left them unable to find time to care for patients' bodies (Picco, Santoro, & Garrino, 2010). Older nurses are embarrassed about their profession on hearing such reports. Conversely, forcing bathing on patients every day is disputed; "bathing people routinely against their wishes—'for their own good'—should become part of nursing history" (Rader et al., 2006, p. 42). Bathing patients ritualistically has been attributed to questionable skin care practices (Skewes, 1996).

In spite of trends in hospital nursing practice where much of hygienic care is delegated to ancillary staff, professional nurses still value the link between bathing and the hygiene of their patients as essential to skin cleanliness, microbiologic safety, and skin health. In one account of a weekend undergraduate nursing program, the faculty and students on a nursing unit bathed all 20 patients to the extreme gratitude of the RNs. RNs are responsible for supervising delegated functions of other nursing staff. RNs recognize that bathing provides an opportunity for skin assessment and the development of a relationship with patients (Freeman, 1997). However, whether the bed bath and other bathing procedures persist as a nursing ritual is debatable. Some nurses reject the notion (Huey, 1986; Huttmann, 1985; Skewes, 1996) that rituals have a place in nursing.

TRADITIONS, BELIEFS, AND DEFINITIONS

Bathing patients is quintessential nursing care (Hektor & Touhy, 1997) and caring for patients' bodies occupies a central role in nursing (Pico et al., 2010). As an example of hands-on, physical care, bathing patients is elemental nursing work (Engebretson, 2002). The cleanliness of patients and the need for nurses to be clean themselves (Smith, 1900a) has been linked historically with nursing in hospitals and with the order and discipline of nursing (Rosenberg, 1987). In the 19th century, hygiene, bathing, and cleanliness were associated with theories of disease and cure; the same principles continue to orient modern nursing (Cayleff, 1987; McGraw & Drennan, 2009; Pipe et al., 2012). According to 19th-century nurses, bathing and washing functioned to keep the body in "proper working order" (Stackpoole, 1889, p. 89). Warm baths were recommended for cleansing and soothing patients (Smith, 1900a, 1900b) and later touted as "one of the most valuable forms of treatment" (Edmonds, 1926, p. 805) that nurses practiced. Changes in patient bathing practices were described, with more active participation of patients expected in the decades following World War II (Sheldon, 1953).

Fundamentals of nursing texts continue to assert that bathing and other hygienic activities result in patients' realizing an improved sense of well-being (Berman, Snyder, & McKinney, 2011; Fuerst & Wolff, 1969; Kozier, Erb, & Olivieri, 1991; Potter & Perry, 2003). The warmth of the bath water is attributed to muscle relaxation and pain relief. Moreover, nurses consider bathing patients to be one of the "good" aspects of care. The bath as an element of morning care, along with other bathing opportunities during a 24-hour hospital day, has allowed nurses to impose order on patient units (Wolf, 1986a, 1989). Bathing patients, as a nursing ritual, may foster healing (Biley & Wright, 1997).

Nurses think that bathing comforts some patients. It is a direct care, hands-on activity (Wolf & Smith, 1997) that is often, but not always, begun after permission is asked. Nurses' hands deliver the cleansing and turning of patients' bodies during bathing. Touching strangers' bodies goes against cultural norms and nurses learn to breach these boundaries. They may assess how bathing and touch are interpreted in the context of patients' cultures and their present situations, then again, they may not. They soon discover that patients and their family members do not always welcome bathing.

Nurses learn to invade patients' personal space when giving hygienic care. They also handle bodily products within this zone of direct care, including excreta and also secretions when caring for infected patients. Nurses, similar to other health care providers, often put their bodies in direct contact with patients' different body parts (Shakespeare, 2003; Twigg, 2002) yet rarely think of their work as embodied.

Students learn the order of washing body parts from the beginning to the end of a complete bath. In this way the bath can be seen as systematic and procedural (Grant, Giddings, & Beale, 2005), even routinized and ritualized. Some parts of the body are cleaner than others, for example, the face and hands are cleaner than the feet, genitals (Gooch, 1989), and perianal skin. This bodywork is private, accomplished "behind the screens" (Lawler, 1991), thereby relegated to nursing's hidden work or taken-for-granted practices (Macleod, 1994).

When the privacy of bathing is interrupted and the threat of patient nudity is real, nurses employed in hospitals and other settings frequently shield patients' bodies from others who may enter patients' rooms or shower rooms, or open curtains. They can use sheets, towels, or blankets to cover patients so that no part of the body is left exposed, close and leave no gaps in the curtain, and restrict other people from entering the room (Downey & Lloyd, 2008). Nurse faculty teach students that the dignity and privacy of patients must be guarded. At the same time they instruct students to encourage patients, as soon as they are judged able, to carry out this care themselves. In this way, patient autonomy and health-promoting agendas are theoretically fostered. Yet, the impulse to bathe all patients at designated times is a significant compulsion for many nurses (Walsh & Ford, 1989). Despite science, the bath has to be done.

When nurses help patients bathe, other activities are accomplished during the nurse–patient interaction. Bathing provides a short time or snapshot to access other patient needs and is a sort of platform for simultaneously achieving nursing activities and obtaining patient requests. Consequently, the patient appreciates skillful nursing care; the patient expresses his or her feelings; and the nurse supports the patient's increasing independence (Taylor, 1994). Nurses' construction of physical and emotional space with patients achieves closeness, necessary to the therapeutic nurse–patient relationship (Savage, 1997). Respect for the patient must always be communicated, as a hospitalized patient's or long-term care resident's sense of well-being is affected during bathing procedures (Wagnild & Manning, 1985).

Nurses' work in acute care and long-term care settings involves direct care of vulnerable people. Why and how nurses are able to perform the care they do is often questioned by outsiders, and sometimes by nurses themselves;

"How can you stand to be a nurse?" By virtue of nursing's access, basic care activities provide an opportunity to pay attention to patients as persons and occasions to create relationships based on trust (Picco et al., 2010). Nurses have continued with caring for the body, and by association give voice to persons ill, diseased, vulnerable, suffering, and marginalized, most often hoping through shared, physical closeness to connect physically, emotionally (Picco et al., 2010), culturally, and even spiritually.

Types of Baths

General hygienic care is performed with or for patients by nursing staff after the patients' condition and ability to perform activities of daily living have been assessed. General hygienic care or total care includes bathing patients' skin and oral hygiene, eye, ear, hair, and nail care. A complete "bed bath" is defined as the nursing intervention of washing a patient's body when he or she requires maximum assistance from nursing staff (Wolf, 1986a). The only body part that patients may be able to wash themselves is their face, but unconscious patients and infants obviously cannot. Traditional bed baths have undergone many changes based on the need for efficiency, control, and research. Some acute care agencies bathe patients with premoistened, no-rinse disposable cloths (Rader et al., 2006) and have introduced bag baths using microwaved, warm, moistened washcloths (Skewes, 1994). In the example of the bag bath, different cloths have been designated for specific areas of the body (Skewes, 1996). Showers or tub baths are often regularly scheduled for residents of long-term care facilities. It is always preferable to continue patients' usual bathing practices (Gooch, 1989) and it is worth taking the time to determine them.

Textbooks, agency procedure manuals, and journal articles specify common equipment assembled for bathing patients (Downey & Lloyd, 2008). Bathing aids such as hydraulic bath chairs and shower chairs help reduce the physical burden for nursing staff. Some of the equipment has been thought to act as infecting agents. For instance, the potential for infection by bath basins ($N = 30$) was examined by Smith, Snedeker, Rivera, Willier, and Mortimer (2012) in a neonatal intensive care unit. They found one or more types of bacteria in 84% of the basins: coagulase-positive *Staphylococcus*, *Corynebacterium* species, *Bacillus* species, and alpha hemolytic *Streptococcus*. Methicillin-resistant *Staphylococcus aureus* (MRSA) was isolated from one basin (5%) and *Pseudomonas aeruginosa* and *Escherichia coli* were isolated from 11% of the basins that grew bacteria.

Patients can participate in a self-help bed bath, also termed *self-care*. They are encouraged to "do" for themselves ideally to foster independence, privacy, and exercise and to hasten healing. Partial or abbreviated baths cleanse parts of patients' bodies that cause discomfort or odor (Berman et al., 2011).

Nurses believe that patients can get better, their conditions will improve, when they bathe themselves (Wolf, 1986a). They encourage patients to care for themselves; they try to capitalize on patients' strengths and participate in making decisions regarding their care. Patients who are able to shower may be bathed sitting on a shower chair, in a tank, or using a Sitz bath. Therapeutic baths or soaks (balneotherapy) are used when large areas of patients' skin are affected; water, saline, colloids, sodium bicarbonate, starch, medicated tars, bath oils, and so forth bring relief to patients suffering from pruritis and dermatologic conditions (Smeltzer, Bare, Hinkle, & Cheever, 2008; Stender, Blichmann, & Serup, 1990). Tepid sponge baths lower temperature of febrile patients by conduction radiation, convection, and evaporation (Pacis, 1986). Certain types of baths have evolved or have been eliminated. For example, an early practice of bathing to raise body temperature to treat syphilis has thankfully been discontinued (Smith, 1936).

BODYWORK AND DIRTY AND CLEAN WORK: POLLUTION AND PURIFICATION

Douglas (1966, 1970, 1975), an anthropologist, provided different ways to understand social attitudes toward people, actions, objects, and work labeled *dirty* by societies. She proposed that in various cultures, a great amount of attention is paid to the demarcation and separation of the sacred and the profane. Not to follow the rituals of separation results in dangerous consequences. Activities that purify (or cleanse) are performed to avert the dangerous effect of breaching the rules and symbolic actions are performed, creating positive effects.

Nursing is a subcultural group in many societies, reflecting the overall, general culture but with distinctions. The ritual behavior demonstrated in bathing practices, in handling potentially dangerous materials such as respiratory secretions, feces, and blood, offer protections to nurses and patients alike. As direct caregivers, nurses and nursing staff handle profane substances routinely, more than other health care providers.

Nursing rituals, such as bathing patients, may dramatize the implicit need of nurses to foster patients' healing and thus are considered therapeutic. On the other hand, keeping patients clean or purifying them day after day, serves as a protection from profane materials including the products of infection. Direct contact with profane substances and the defiled or abjected (Holmes, Perron, & O'Byrne, 2006) members of social groups, such as persons with AIDS, is greatly feared by many in society. To manage this work, nurses rely on rituals, governed by policies, procedures, and routines. As such contact is part of accepted nursing work, nurses strive to protect patients from stigma.

Nurses' contacts with sexual organs, including the breasts, vagina, penis, and testes, link nurses with perceptions of prostitution in male fantasy (Twigg, 2000) and potentially implies someone involved in immoral activities. Nurses are aware of these stereotypes. When patients seem to act out sexually during hygienic care, for example by seeming to enjoy genital exposure, nurses pass on this information often during change-of-shift reports. In this way, patient behavior is punished typically by avoidance or perhaps directly in conversation. Deeper motivations explaining the behavior may or may not be evaluated.

Nurses are judged to be polluted by direct contact with sexual organs, contact with naked bodies, profane substances, and marginalized people. They can be perceived as dirty workers (Tyndale, 1992). Because of this proximity with patients, residents, and community members in close, personal space, they have extraordinary status issues in society (Davis, 1984). Nurses can experience occupational stigma and are discredited by some. Society is ambivalent about nursing, and nursing work is consequently undermined or destabilized (Twigg, 2002) owing to bodywork. Since much of nursing work is private, hidden work by virtue of the need to protect patients' privacy and dignity, and imperative for all nurses to follow for tending to all patients, including the marginalized, ill, deformed, and imperfect, and, contain profane materials, nursing's knowledge is often invisible. Twigg (2000) and others have suggested that nursing is ambivalent about its performance of bodywork; they have argued that the emphasis on high-tech interventions and machines (clean work), psychological dimensions of patients (emphasis on caring work), and "academicizing" (conceptual and theoretical work) nursing represents "a further flight from the bodily in pursuit of higher status forms of knowledge and practice" (p. 399).

Nursing's clean work and dirty work are intertwined with its societal role. Cleanliness, for nurses and patients, is part of nursing's propaganda for achieving wellness. Cleanliness accomplishes practical and scientific outcomes. Intimate care during caring moments in caring situations provides a platform to preach, teach, or promote the value of good hygiene and the benefits of self-care. Nurses typically have more time than other health care providers with patients, and can use their presence to advantage.

Nurses' freedom to access patients' bodies (Picco et al., 2010) is a gift. They learn about patients' bodies, everyday lives, suffering, families, and friends and about themselves; they grow through reflective experience. They witness and experience magical, spiritual, moral, and ethical aspects of life and confront many complex dilemmas of the people they serve (Wolf, 1986b). Following Florence Nightingale's lead, nurses have been urged to consider their profession as moral and sacred: "No task is holier or more sacred than that of ministering to the sick" (Talcott, 1895, p. 31). As a vocation and a profession, nurses have been admonished to consider what they do as more than just a job, but as a calling. This perspective may not be held by every nurse today.

INITIATION TO BATHING PATIENTS

Some initiation into this part of a nurse's work is evident. Nursing students prepare to bathe or assist patients with bathing and other types of intimate care through simulated experiences, student-centered methods, or more traditional approaches (Jeffries, Rew, & Cramer, 2002). As they begin clinical experiences, they are vulnerable when thinking about how they will carry out fundamental care of patients (Grant et al., 2005). When confronting the challenge of moving into patients' personal space and touching their bodies, including the very private body parts of patients of a gender different from their own, students are often anxious and fear that they may harm patients. They are surprised that patients help them get through the experience; students are self-conscious, concerned with privacy, and increasingly confident as the bathing progresses (Wolf, 1997). Their initiation into basic nursing care may or may not be witnessed by clinical faculty; they are often alone with patients when performing intimate care.

Lawler (1991) noted that nurses' experiences of learning body care have not been well researched. The "breaking of social norms which many nursing acts involve...they learn through experience" (p. 119). Lawler identified the terror, embarrassment, and timidity felt when nurses undress patients. Berry (1986) shared that:

> *We are taught the proper way to carry out a bed bath, but not how to deal with the breaking of the social taboos when we wash a patient's body. Most nurses remember the fear they felt when doing their first bed bath. As a young female you work with a patient (who might well be male), behind drawn curtains and are expected to strip and wash his whole body. I remember feeling shamed and confused; my hands felt stiff, cold, awkward and useless. A bed bath can be embarrassing for the patient at the best of time but far worse when the nurse herself is embarrassed. (p. 56)*

The task of touching patients' bodies, specifically to bathe them, may initially violate nursing students' social and cultural taboos (Grant et al., 2005). This becomes even more complicated; in spite of religious or cultural restrictions, some male or female students must perform the bath as part of the experiential transition to the professional role.

Although nursing students' initiation is relatively unsupported by clinical faculty, they nonetheless manage to cope with intimate bodily care. On the other hand, many nursing faculty have created safe zones for students to share some of the contradictions and tensions associated with this type of bodywork. One example is faculty who use reflective practice to examine the everyday nursing practice of giving a bath. In this case, the student helped a patient experience an immersion bath and detailed her reflections on the experience. She used "reflection on action" to examine the experience (O'Regan & Fawcett, 2006).

A nurse has doubted the nursing faculty's commitment to teaching fundamental skills because they are thought to be less complex than other course content and skills. She questions how RNs can adequately supervise NAs if they do not learn or practice basic skills themselves (Pasquale, 2008).

Nurses are also initiated into more complex bathing practices as they progress in their careers. More seasoned nurses show them the way. They learn to bathe patients in severe pain, with many tubes, with traumatic injuries, who are older, unconscious, and who have suffered strokes, myocardial infarction, burns, and acute renal failure. In this way, they may unconsciously adopt the techniques of the body displayed by other nurses, with their developing skills and relationships with patients very similar to those whom they emulated (Savage, 1997).

THE ART OF BATHING PATIENTS

Knowing how to bathe patients so that direct care performance is perceived as an art requires a great deal of clinical practice; nursing art is developed gradually. The art of nursing includes nurses' direct understanding of situations, their intuitive and embodied knowing that comes from the practice of nursing (Chinn, 1994); artistic nurses know what is created in the acts of direct nursing care, such as bathing patients. Artistic performance of nursing care for complex patients is not captured nor necessarily witnessed. Some experts may be truly superior at caring for difficult, challenging patients. Nurses who excel at this skill often mentor others' performance. Other colleagues recognize their excellence.

In one example of such mentorship, a seasoned nurse taught a new graduate nurse how to clean a patient with cancer and extensive bony metastasis after her third episode of diarrhea that evening. The expert nurse participated in and directed the less experienced, recent graduate to move the patient, contain the diarrhea, speak to the patient, gently wash her body, and place linens in anticipation of the next diarrheal episode, initiating the neophyte into more skilled practices for bathing such a challenging patient (Wolf, 1986a). "Skill in bathing patients increased...and was gained when a neophyte worked with a skilled, seasoned nurse" (p. 374).

Nurses who are skilled artists are viewed by patients as conscientious and very careful. They make them comfortable, explain things well, acknowledge patients' responsibilities in self-care, soothe the body through hands-on skills, and spend time with patients to plan care. They also give confidence back to patients and relieve their pain (Taylor, 1994). A patient shared her views:

> What I liked about the bath was it was hot. It took the pain away. It made me sleepy. I feel Sue's [the nurse] begun to give me a bit of confidence back. I don't really know. She makes me feel that I am going to get better. I can do things. (p. 166)

Her nurse used the bath as a "mechanism" to help her accept additional holistic therapies so that she could perform other bodywork, such as massage, to release her negative feelings, so the bath was a medium for other therapeutic agents.

> It worked out well. [T]he other thing about today's bath is that she was very down beforehand. She said to me: "I can't get anything right"...but afterwards she was very positive. (Taylor, 1994, p. 166)

A more recent example of bathing that is artistic has been developed by colleagues challenged with bathing individuals with dementia in a person-directed way. Rader and colleagues (2006) have conceptualized bathing as a human interaction, not a task, and a pleasant experience. They investigated person-centered bathing methods aimed at meeting the needs and comfort levels of nursing-home residents and at reducing their discomfort, agitation, and aggression. Furthermore, they considered bathing patients against their wishes as abuse, unless a health reason necessitated it. They identified negative reactions of dementia patients to routine showering in long-term care facilities and helped nurses and certified NAs evaluate such behavioral symptoms as expressions of unmet needs. Nursing staff learned communication techniques and problem-solving approaches to identify causes of behavioral manifestations and potential solutions. They adapted the environment to residents' comfort and security. Staff learned that focusing on the person and relationship reduced discomfort and behavioral symptoms. They worked with rather than against resistance.

Covering patients with a towel and washing beneath it, medicating patients with routine analgesia for musculoskeletal problems, using hot packs for sore joints before a bath, moving limbs carefully, being aware of discomfort, and encouraging residents to participate in bathing comprised recommendations. Using no-rinse products, padding shower chairs or using padded chairs with foot support, and enlisting family members in bathing may also help, and commercial bath-in-a-bag products or baths-in-a-bag made at home were also advocated. The person-directed care of individuals with dementia is detailed in a CD-ROM and book (Barrick, Rader, Hoeffer, Sloane, & Biddle, 2008).

Bathing disability, the inability to wash and dry one's whole body without personal assistance, is another phenomenon of concern to nurses and other health care professionals who have assessed elderly persons' gradual loss of autonomy with performance of activities of daily living and as a mark of their frailty (Rozzini, Sabatini, Ranhoff, & Trabucchi, 2007). Investigators have studied instrumental activities of daily living (using the telephone, preparing meals, doing housework, taking medicines, and handling money), activities of daily living (bathing, dressing, transferring from bed to chair, using a toilet, and eating), and other risk factors to predict new-onset disability (Mehta et al., 2011). Bathing disability is linked to admission to long-term care facilities and labeled a sentinel event for older persons, even predicting subsequent disability (Gill, Guo, & Allore, 2006) and death.

Bathing disability suggests a need for nurses to investigate older persons' ability to self-bathe during bathing episodes. Many of the oldest old require help with bathing (Berlau, Corrada, Peltz, & Kawas, 2011). Nurses in hospitals might determine best practices to help older persons reduce the progression of bathing disability using specific interventions. In addition, encouraging long-term care residents to bathe themselves partially helps them maintain some independence (Ahluwalia, Gill, Baker, & Fried, 2010).

The evolution of bathing techniques, equipment, patient approaches, and research evidence the transformation of the nursing ritual of bathing patients. Bathing is part of nursing practices that address the control of dangerous materials, such as infectious secretions or excretions. Bathing may also be an occupational ritual or ritual of transition whereby a nursing student learns the role of the nurse.

RESEARCH ON BATHING AND HYGIENIC INTERVENTIONS

The citations in Table 2.1 comprise a selection of texts addressing bathing in the context of nursing care. The literature reviewed is research; investigators used quantitative and qualitative approaches to sample nurses, NAs, and patients involved in bathing activities. These publications demonstrate a more than 50-year concern of professional nursing with bathing patients, hygienic practices, and infection control. Combined with historic antecedents on maintaining cleanliness and assuring personal hygiene that goes back to before the turn of the 19th century, this literature shows nursing's commitment to the care of patients.

BATHS, BATHING, AND SYMBOLS

The details on how to give patients a traditional bed bath in hospitals are readily available on the web via YouTube (Hawknurse, 2008), accessible to many, and perhaps relegating bathing to what is termed *secular* or *lay knowledge*. However, bathing patients represents more latent or symbolic meanings for professional nurses. Nurses own hygienic care. They handle both the sacred and the profane of human life as they work.

As nurses lay hands on one to cleanse, comfort, and heal, they accomplish many agendas for patients and themselves. By virtue of this private work, they implicitly wash away disease and impose order and control on unit activities ("At least the bath is done!"). Not bathing patients suggests disorder. Traditionally, there have been scheduled bathing opportunities on every shift, again exacting some kind of social control. This type of order helps establish certainty on acute care units where uncertainty is the norm and patients often rapidly "go bad" and need to be rescued.

Despite the associated status issues with being dirty workers (Lawler, 1991), handling excreta and secretions and control of these products as well as products of infection are an important part of nurses' work. They attempt to keep clean and dirty separate through infection control practices and in the way they use space, the architecture of the agencies in which they work, equipment, and personal protections. The nursing imperative is to keep patients

TABLE 2.1
Reviewed Citations

Study/Article	Theoretical Basis for Study	Design; Question/Purpose; Sampling Frame/Size	Independent Variables (IV); Dependent Variables (DV)	Measurement of Variables (Name of Instrument, etc.)	Statistics Used to Answer Research Question	Findings
Winslow, Lane, and Gaffney (1985)	Physiologic: oxygen consumption, heart rate, and rate pressure product correlate with myocardial oxygen consumption	Quasi-experimental; to compare oxygen uptake and cardiovascular responses in control and acute myocardial infarction adult patient during bathing (basin bath, tub bath, and shower); adult patients (n = 17 postmyocardial infarction and n = 22 control subjects)	Physiologic responses (peak heart rate, rate pressure product, oxygen consumption) (DV) before, during and after three types of baths (basin, tub, and shower) (IV)	Peak heart rate (Holter monitor electrocardiogram), cuff sphygmomanometer, rate pressure product, oxygen consumption (open circuit, indirect calorimetry); perceived exertion (Borg); ranks of appropriateness of type of bath at patients' stage of recovery	Three-way analysis of variance (group by sex by activity type) with repeated measures over one factor (activity type: rest, basin bath, tub bath, and shower)	No significant differences in oxygen consumption between controls and patients at rest; female patients had significantly higher heart rate and rate pressure product than control females. During bathing, male and female patients had significantly lower oxygen consumption and higher peak heart rates and rate pressure products than controls. Physiologic costs of three types of baths are similar
Parsons, Peard, and Page (1985)	Physiologic mechanisms	Quasi-experimental; to investigate the effects of three nursing hygiene interventions (oral care, body hygiene, indwelling catheter care) on the cerebrovascular status of severe closed head injured persons; severe closed head injured persons (N = 14 or 15) in surgical intensive care unit	Nursing hygiene interventions (oral care, body hygiene, indwelling catheter care) (IV); cerebrovascular status (DV)	DV: MICP, MABP, HR, CPP, and temperature	Analysis of variance; two-way analysis of variance	All hygiene interventions caused significant increases in HR, MABP, MICP, and CPP

Wolf (1986a)	Frame of reference: anthropological, sociological, and nursing literature	Context: medical nursing unit in large urban hospital to study (a) postmortem care, (b) admission of patients to the hospital and discharge of patients from the hospital, (c) medication administration, (d) bath, handling of excreta and secretions, caring for patients with infectious disease, and (e) change-of-shift report	Participant observation (fieldwork) and field notes, semistructured interviews, event analysis, document analysis	Therapeutic nursing ritual: the bath, bathing patients; postmortem care (context do not resuscitate dilemma); medication administration
	What actions, words, and objects make up nursing rituals?			Occupational nursing ritual: change-of-shift report
	What are the types of nursing rituals demonstrated by professional nurse caring for adult patients?			Patient ritual: admission to the hospital
	What explicit or manifest meanings do these rituals have to nurses, patients, and their families, and to other hospital personnel?			Bath: nurses bathed patients frequently; often the same patient may have been bathed during each shift. Nurses considered the hygiene of their patients to be their domain. The control of patients' hygiene through the bath, their handling of excreta and secretions, their repeated washings of patients, and their ability to be in direct contact with infected patients exposed on a symbolic level how the maintenance of cleanliness achieved order in a place that could easily become disordered
	What implicit or latent meanings are identified by the nurses, patients, and other hospital personnel, and by the investigator?			
	How do nursing rituals emerge in the content of postmortem care, medication administration, admission and discharge procedures, change-of-shift report, and the aseptic practices of nurses, including the bed bath and the care of infected patients?			
	Informants: nurses, patients, family members, hospital personnel			

(continued)

TABLE 2.1
Reviewed Citations (continued)

Study/ Article	Theoretical Basis for Study	Design; Question/Purpose; Sampling Frame/Size	Independent Variables (IV); Dependent Variables (DV)	Measurement of Variables (Name of Instrument, etc.)	Statistics Used to Answer Research Question	Findings
Hardy (1990)	Physiologic factors placing elderly at risk for dry skin	Quasi-experimental; repeated measures (9 data points); to isolate clinical indicators of dry skin in the elderly, test an instrument to measure dry skin, analyze the importance of factors thought to contribute to dry skin, test the importance of factors thought to contribute to dry skin, and determine the feasibility of clinical implementation of protocol; elderly residents of long-term care facility with nursing and medical diagnosis of dry skin ($N = 15$)	Skin condition: etiologic factors, skin condition (redness, scaling, fissuring, rash, excoriation, greasy appearance, thickening). DV: bathing protocol; use of superfatted soap (Dove) for cleansing; water temperature of 90°F–100°F; immerse in tub up to chest pouring water over body parts not immersed or shower with continuous spray over all body parts for 10 minutes; pat, rather than rub, the skin dry with a cotton towel; apply mineral oil over all body parts; wear cotton clothing	Modified version of SCDF	Multivariate analysis of variance	Mean dryness scores decreased during intervention and returned to baseline when intervention discontinued (redness, scaling, flaking)

| Lawler (1991) | Grounded theory: Theory arises from ordinary everyday business of nursing social life; ethnomethodology: ways (strategies) nurses make lives manageable and meaningful; Garfinkel's notion of disrupted social order | Qualitative, grounded theory; to examine nurses' socialization about the body; interviewees ($N = 34$), 27 RNs, 2 students, 5 enrolled nurses | How nurses overcome what they have been socialized to believe about the body, body exposure, and body accessibility in our culture; what thy remember of the first time they performed body care for another; what occupationally specific methods they learn that facilitate doing their work, especially those aspects that are invasive of the body and therefore give rise to potential and actual embarrassment; how the context of care is constructed so that it is socially permissible to touch the body to provide nursing care; how nurses negotiate the social territory of doing for patients what they would normally do for themselves in private; how they manage when they must touch those parts of body that are proscribed, and how they construct these encounters with patients so that this level of intimacy is possible; how they manage sexuality and sexual behavior during body care, and what they do when the situation becomes problematic; how they manage the body care of dying patients and the dead body; how they care for others when the tasks to be performed are potentially or | Observational data, field notes, semistructured interviews | Grounded theory and ethnomethodology methods | How nurses manage the body: The body and nursing, conceptualizing the body, social life and the body; the body and sexuality. Somological practice: body care and learning to do for others, embarrassment, social rules, and the context of body care; the body, illness experience, and nursing; the body in recovery, dying, and death; sexuality, the body, and nursing; Theory of somology |

(continued)

TABLE 2.1
Reviewed Citations (continued)

Study/ Article	Theoretical Basis for Study	Design; Question/Purpose; Sampling Frame/Size	Independent Variables (IV): Dependent Variables (DV)	Measurement of Variables (Name of Instrument, etc.)	Statistics Used to Answer Research Question	Findings
			actually nauseating, or truly awful; how they help people cope with a dysfunctional, disfigured, deformed, or damaged body in illness experience; how they recognize embarrassment and manage it; how they purposefully and deliberatively help patients with situations that would generally be considered embarrassing; how patients make the nurse's job easier or more difficult during body care, and what particular patient behaviors facilitate or hamper the nurse's activities; how they manage an occupation that concerns aspects of life normally kept from public view and not discussed openly, and which may be considered dirty or sexual; how they manage nursing care of the body when the patient has a high public profile or high status			

Robichaud-Ekstrand (1991)	Effect of low-workload activity on cardiac physiologic indicators and subjective exertion. Bathing methods' scores (HR, mean blood pressure, rate–pressure product, perceived exertion) higher than prebathing resting scores	Experimental, to compare the effects of a sitting shower versus sitting sink bath in low-risk patients with myocardial infarction on HR, mean blood pressure and rate–pressure product, perceived exertion, and symptoms; within-subject design with randomized counterbalancing of order of baths; low-risk patients ($N = 30$) with myocardial infarction	Shower versus sitting sink self-bath (IV); mean HR, blood pressure, rate–pressure product; perceived exertion; occurrence of symptoms during baths and between resting, bathing, and recovery periods	Analysis of variance and Tukey HSD post hoc test; Friedman test; Wilcoxin post hoc pairwise tests; Pearson rho correlations	Significant differences in activity states (pretest, bathing methods, posttest) for HR, mean blood pressure, rate–pressure product; no significant differences between sitting sink bath and sitting shower
Campbell and Illingworth (1992)	Wetting treated skin increases the severity of skin reaction; soap and friction caused by washing and drying damages the skin	Quasi-experimental, to compare severity of skin reaction to breast and skin wall when not washing, washing with water alone, or washing with soap and water; patients receiving adjuvant radiotherapy to breast or chest wall ($N = 95$)	Washing policies (IV); bolus and no bolus groups (vaseline, not vaseline) (IV); subjective and measurements of acute skin reactions (DV)	Washing policies: not washing; washing with water alone, washing with soap and water (IV); bolus and no bolus groups (IV); subjective (symptoms of itching and pain); objective (erythema; desquamation) measurements of acute skin reactions	T-test most likely	Little difference between washing with water alone and washing with soap and water; skin reactions were less frequent if patients were washing

(continued)

43

TABLE 2.1
Reviewed Citations (continued)

Study/ Article	Theoretical Basis for Study	Design; Question/Purpose; Sampling Frame/Size	Independent Variables (IV); Dependent Variables (DV)	Measurement of Variables (Name of Instrument, etc.)	Statistics Used to Answer Research Question	Findings
Allison, Miller, Squires, and Gau (1993)	Circulating catecholamine associated with cardiac arrhythmias and myocardial ischemia in patients with coronary artery disease also increased during heat stress and moderately intense or prolonged exercise	Quasi-experimental, to assess the safety of hot tub use for men with stable coronary artery disease by determining changes in body temperature, cardiovascular stress, and circulating catecholamines during immersion in hot tub and to compare responses in hot tub to those after 15 minutes of exercise on cycle ergometer at standard prescribed exercise; men with coronary artery disease ($N = 15$)	Hot tub use versus pedaling on cycle ergometer (IV); body temperature, cardiovascular stress, circulating catecholamines, subjective comfort, symptoms (DV)	DV: tympanic temperature, skin temperature, electrocardiographic findings, blood pressure, comfort or perceived exertion ratings (Comfort Index), symptoms (shortness of breath, chest pain, nausea, light-headedness, drowsiness, overheating; scale), free epinephrine and norepinephrine	One-way analysis of variance (baseline to 15 minutes of immersion versus exercise)	Cardiovascular stress of hot tub usage is mild and significantly less stressful than exercise; there may be adequate cardiac output and coronary perfusion during immersion in hot tub

44

Author	Purpose	Design/Sample	Measures	Instruments	Findings
Kovach and Meyer-Arnold (1996)	To examine behaviors of clients with cognitive impairment during bath time and to compare the experiences of tub, bath, and shower. Environmental factors and caregiver behaviors associated with the initiation of aggressive behaviors and activity disturbances were examined	Qualitative, to examine behaviors of clients with cognitive impairment during bath time and to compare experiences of tub, bath, and shower; nonparticipant observation on attendees at adult day care program or residents of special care unit at one facility ($N = 33$)	Behaviors of clients with cognitive impairment during bath time; compare experiences of tub, bath, and shower	Data collection sheets to record subject behavior, caregiver behavior, events or changes in environment	Calm or agitated behaviors were global attributes of subjects' behaviors. Baths/showers were confusing, fearful, and sometimes uncomfortable experiences; subjects did not want to be receiving personal hygiene care but were overpowered by verbal and physical directives of caregiver. Initiating the bathing experience involves an invasion of cognitively impaired subjects' personal reality as well as an invasion of the subject's personal body space

(continued)

TABLE 2.1
Reviewed Citations (continued)

Study/Article	Theoretical Basis for Study	Design; Question/Purpose; Sampling Frame/Size	Independent Variables (IV); Dependent Variables (DV)	Measurement of Variables (Name of Instrument, etc.)	Statistics Used to Answer Research Question	Findings
Wolf (1997)	Bathing patients tacitly incorporated into nursing's identity	Qualitative; to describe nursing students' experiences bathing an adult patient for the first time; phenomenologic; junior nursing students (N = 16)	Experiences bathing an adult patient for the first time	Written responses to question: Tell me what it was like to bathe your first patient		Stressful and challenging experience; avoided performing the bath; were uncomfortable about bathing a stranger; felt clumsy; wanted to avoid causing harm to patient; open to patients' situations and their discomfort; discomfort decreased as the bath progressed
Hartig (1998)	To understand NA actions: types of activities	Qualitative: descriptive naturalistic inquiry, to elicit NA's descriptions of their care activities to understand their contributions to resident care, limitation of the NA role; purposive sample, expert NAs (N = 8) in nursing home	Type of care activities performed by NAs	Face-to-face, semistructured interviews: how do you as an NA contribute to resident care? Describe different types of care you give		Functional care activities (activities of daily living including bathing, etc.; instrumental activities of daily living); psychosocial care activities; delegated care activities

Citation	Purpose	Design/Sample	Variables	Instruments	Analysis	Findings
Hancock, Bowman, and Prater (2000)	Difference in impressions between current and soft towel bed-bathing methods; difference in cost between both methods	Comparative descriptive study, to compare soft towel bed-bathing method with current bed-bathing method on patient satisfaction, nursing staff satisfaction/ acceptance, and costs (labor/materials); medical and surgical patients ($n = 200$); trainee nurses ($n = 200$)	Bed-bathing method (current & soft towel [Toffman: Whitley Industries with Dermalux solution]) (IV); impressions (DV); cost (DV)	Questionnaires: patient (seven questions: privacy, skin warmth, skin cleanliness, skin dryness, skin softness, comfort, relaxing), nurse (eight questions: learning, performing, patient contact, patient feedback, cleanliness, dry hands, soft hands) semistructured interviews (overall impressions of bed-bathing method); cost (solution/ soap, water, electricity, laundry, waste, labor)	Chi-squared test for independence	Patients: Statistically significant differences on skin softness, comfort, relaxation; nurses with more positive responses on soft towel bed bath: statistically significant differences on learning, performing, patient contact, patient feedback, cleanliness, dry hands, and soft hands and very high acceptance for soft towel method

(continued)

TABLE 2.1
Reviewed Citations (continued)

Study/ Article	Theoretical Basis for Study	Design; Question/Purpose; Sampling Frame/Size	Independent Variables (IV); Dependent Variables (DV)	Measurement of Variables (Name of Instrument, etc.)	Statistics Used to Answer Research Question	Findings
Larson et al. (2004)	Infection control: Skin microbial counts and other outcomes when types of baths compared	Quasi-experimental; to compare traditional basin bed bath with prepackaged disposable bed bath on outcomes: time and quality of bath, microbial counts on skin, nurses' satisfaction, and costs; acutely ill patients in intensive care units (N = 40)	To compare traditional basin bath with prepackaged disposable bath (Comfort Bath, Sage Products Inc., Cary, IL) (IV); time, quality of bath, microbial counts on skin, nurses' satisfaction, costs (DV)	Microbiologic sampling; one side of groin and area around umbilicus swabbed and plated; total counts obtained and counts of gram-negative rods; time and quality of bath; time of baths (stopwatch); nurses' satisfaction (interview); costs of bath types (direct product charges, cost of nurses' time, laundry costs) measured	Chi-squared test and Fisher exact test compared quality indicators between traditional and disposable bath; paired *t*-test compared mean bath times; paired *t*-test compared mean log bacterial counts on colonies before and after each type of bath and between traditional and disposable baths; analysis of variance compared bathing time for traditional	Differences in skin microbiology (total bacterial counts) for patients bathed with two different methods were not clinically significantly at groin or periumbilical site; nurses preferred the disposable bath and time for gathering bath supplies was significantly shorter. When nurses' time was considered, costs for traditional and disposable baths were comparable

| | | | | | bath between patients whose bath water was changed and patients whose bath water was not changed. Denominators varied for products used in cost analysis |
| Lomborg, Bjørn, Dahl, and Kirkevold (2005) | Symbolic interaction: APBC; lived body of persons with chronic, serious illness | Qualitative, grounded theory; to explore patients' experiences of being assisted with personal body care; convenience sample (N = 12) patients with severe chronic obstructive lung disease | How patients with COPD perceive personal body care; what it is like to be assisted with personal body care in a hospital setting under circumstances of dependency caused primarily by breathlessness; how patients manage the performance of APBD | Bathing sessions: participant observation; in-depth interviews; field notes; measurement of perceived breathlessness before and after APBC (Modified 1–10 Borg Scale) | Grounded theory methods | Patients were: Struggling for self-preservation (a threefold strategy with inherent dilemmas); not letting go (stoical suffering; enduring; using personal body care as a means to preserve integrity); coping with dependency (realizing and accepting dependency; being a "good" patient; justifying one's needs); minimizing the risk of escalating breathlessness. APBC is complex for hospitalized patients; symbolic and practical necessity for preserving personal integrity and their dependency |

(continued)

TABLE 2.1
Reviewed Citations (continued)

Study/ Article	Theoretical Basis for Study	Design; Question/Purpose; Sampling Frame/Size	Independent Variables (IV); Dependent Variables (DV)	Measurement of Variables (Name of Instrument, etc.)	Statistics Used to Answer Research Question	Findings
Lomborg and Kirkevold (2005)	APBC	Qualitative, grounded theory; to present professional nursing challenges in providing care to patients suffering from COPD on nurses' expectations, goals, and approaches to APBC; cases of nurse–patient interactions in APBC ($N = 12$) patients hospitalized with severe COPD	How can APBC be characterized in hospitalized patients with severe COPD? What are the main problem(s) in completing APBC; How do nurses deal with the professional challenge of providing assistance?	Bathing sessions: participant observation; semistructured interviews with patients (background experiences of living with COPD; experiences of being a patient receiving nursing care); observed APBC sessions; semistructured interviews with nurses, followed by in-depth interviews; Modified Borg Scale: measure patients' perceived breathlessness before and after APBC; textual notes recorded	Grounded theory principles	Curtailing process: mutual, dynamic process during APBC; depended on the integrated competencies of nurses; components and dimensions of curtailing the APBC to meet needs of patients suffering from severe COPD: Breathlessness—a basic premise; essential curtailing acts (activities related to patients' bodies; partial body care; pauses; instruction and information elements; attached elements); economizing the patient's energy; creating an atmosphere conducive of curtailing dimensions: recognition of patients' breathing difficulties; carrying out essential curtailing acts; economizing patients' energy; creating an atmosphere conducive of curtailing

| Mahoney, Trudeau, Penyack, and MacLeod (2006) | Intervention research: delivery (primarily actions of interventionist); receipt (client knowledge and skill); enactment (factors in naturalistic setting that affect clients' ability to carry out the intervention); origins of behavioral symptoms; resistiveness to care | Qualitative: descriptive; secondary analysis of field data using content analysis, to analyze intervention implementation issues encountered within the bathing persons with Alzheimer's disease at home (BATH) study; personal caring at home; (N = 42 care recipient–caregiver dyads); 130 home intervention visits (clients with Alzheimer's disease) | Analyze intervention implementation issues encountered within the BATH study | Direct observation, field notes recorded immediately following home visits, caregiver journal data, transcribed notes from researcher and caregiver-initiated telephone calls and team meetings | Intervention delivery required a nurse interventionist trained thoroughly in protocols and could implement them rigorously to maintain intervention, integrity, was knowledgeable about special issues with the study population, and flexible and able to form a partnership with the caring dyad. Delivery of tailored intervention depended on assessment of care recipient and caregiver behavior; receipt of intervention influenced by factors within person, relationship, and interaction; application of intervention overlaps previous issues affecting delivery and receipt; caregiver perceptions of efficacy recorded in journals impacted caregiver practices essential to learning new skill and applying them when nurse interventions not in home; five key lessons identified |

(continued)

TABLE 2.1
Reviewed Citations (continued)

Study/Article	Theoretical Basis for Study	Design; Question/Purpose; Sampling Frame/Size	Independent Variables (IV); Dependent Variables (DV)	Measurement of Variables (Name of Instrument, etc.)	Statistics Used to Answer Research Question	Findings
Lomborg and Kirkevold (2007)	Symbolic interaction: elements required to facilitate effective cooperation between nurses and patients during body care (washing and bathing); includes reaching a common situation, negotiating a common scope and structure, and clarifying rules	Qualitative, grounded theory; to explore patients' experiences of being assisted with personal body care; cases of nurse–patient interactions in APBC ($N = 12$) patients hospitalized with severe COPD	Nurse–patient interactions in APBC	Participants' experiences analyzed to understand actions observed from perspective of the experiences: bathing sessions; observation; field notes; audio recordings	Grounded theory methods	Achieving therapeutic clarity: Nurses and patients have different expectations and worked toward different goals in body care sessions. Major barriers to achieving therapeutic clarity: Reaching a common understanding of the patient's current condition and stage of illness trajectory; negotiating a common scope and structuring body care sessions; clarifying roles

Source	Purpose	Design/Sample	Bathing description	Methods	Findings
Happ, Tate, Swigart, DiVirgilio-Thomas, and Hoffman (2010)	Physiologic research on effects of bathing on oxygen consumption	Secondary analysis of microethnographic study, to describe practices and beliefs about bathing patients during weaning during prolonged mechanical ventilation; purposive sampling ($N = 30$) adult patients during weaning from prolonged mechanical ventilation	Bathing activities (no protocols on type of bed bath, bath-in-a-bag or basin with water) during ventilator weaning trials regarding the optimal timing and importance of bathing; need to reduce energy demands during weaning	Field notes and interviews analyzed using grounded theory analytic techniques; hygiene included reference to personal care, cleaning, bathing, and dressing changes	Hygienic care associated with attentiveness, caring and "good" nursing care. Personal and social value of bathing; ambiguity and contradiction about effects of bathing on patients who are undergoing weaning trials; working weaning trials around the bath; and recognizing individual patient response to bathing
Ahluwalia et al. (2010)	Self-care performance of activities of daily living, specifically bathing; to explore and understand bathing experience from the perspective of older persons	Qualitative, grounded theory; to explore and understand the bathing experience from the perspective of older persons by describing their practices, preferences, and goals regarding the bathing task; ($N = 23$) community-living persons	In-depth, semistructured interviews: descriptions of childhood and current bathing habits, meaning and purpose of bathing, difficulties and concerns about bathing, goals of and preferences for independent bathing, and use of and attitude toward different types of bathing assistance	Grounded theory methods: coding scheme, axial coding, categories, triangulation with quantitative data in larger study	Themes: importance and significance of bathing; variability in attitudes, preferences and sources of bathing assistance; anticipation of and responses to bathing disability

(continued)

53

TABLE 2.1
Reviewed Citations (continued)

Study/ Article	Theoretical Basis for Study	Design; Question/Purpose; Sampling Frame/Size	Independent Variables (IV); Dependent Variables (DV)	Measurement of Variables (Name of Instrument, etc.)	Statistics Used to Answer Research Question	Findings
Jury, Gierrero, Burant, Cadnum, and Donskey (2011)	Efficacy of bathing for removal of *Clostridium difficile* spores from *C. difficile* infected patients' skin and tested whether showers were more effective than bed baths for removal of spores. Determined frequency and type of bathing performed; identified factors that limited patients' ability to bathe	Prospective cohort study, to evaluate efficacy of bathing for removal of *C. difficile* spores for patients with *C. difficile* infection and determine if showers are more effective than baths for removal of spores; hospitalized and long-term care patients (N = 74)	Type of bath, shower versus bed bath (IV); *C. difficile* skin culture results for abdomen, chest, forearm, hand, groin	Medical record review; questionnaire to determine bathing practices (frequency and type (shower or bed bath); factors limiting ability to bathe; mobility score; odor and appearance of colonies and positive reaction using *C. difficile* latex agglutination assay; in vivo toxin production using *C. difficile* Tox A/B II	Cochran Q, repeated measures, compared proportions of positive hand-imprint culture results before and after bathing; *t*-test compared mean number of colonies acquired on hands before and after bathing; repeated measures 2 × 2 analysis of variance tested differences in number of colonies before and after bathing for each skin site cultured	Quality and frequency of bathing of patients with *C. difficile* in agency limited by decreased mobility, presence of devices, and pain; showering associated with significant decrease in frequency and mean number of spores acquired on hands

| O'Horo, Silva, Munoz-Price, and Safdar (2012) | Assess efficacy of daily bathing with CHG for prevention of health care-associated BSIs | Systematic review and meta-analysis of randomized controlled trials and quasi-experimental studies | 1 randomized controlled trial and 11 nonrandomized controlled trials | Independent data extraction of over six databases/other resources by three authors; PRISMA flow diagram used to present study selection process | Pooled odds ratio using random-effects model was 0.44 (95% CI, 0.33,0.59, $p < .00001$) | Daily bathing with CHG reduced incidence of BSIs, including central line-associate BSIs among medical ICU patients |

APBC, assisted personal body care; BSI, bloodstream infection; CHG, chlorhexidine; COPD, chronic obstructive pulmonary disease; CPP, cerebral perfusion pressure; HR, heart rate; MABP, mean arterial blood pressure; MICP, mean intracranial pressure; NA, nursing assistant; SCDM, Skin Condition Data Form.

clean. Nurses may sanction other nurses who leave a patient incontinent for more than 15 minutes, most often during the change-of-shift report.

Emergency nurses at the frontline of patient admissions to acute care agencies care for patients who are considered unclean by society or by virtue of soiling during vehicular and workplace accidents. They are the first in line to cleanse patients, to make them more approachable for care by health care providers. When patients' body odors are intense, nurses work diligently to improve this. Consequently and practically, bathing patients not only eases the access of health care providers to patients, but symbolically purifies them.

Gloves, universal precautions, high-impact interventions (Collins, 2010), isolation procedures, and meticulous hand hygiene are used to protect nurses and patients from infecting organisms. They attempt to protect all in their places of work from contamination and infection. In this way, nursing body-work can be seen as dangerous work. Research literature on the need for basic care, illustrated by the connection of oral care with ventilator-acquired pneumonia, has proliferated along with a focus by patient safety committees, health care providers, and hospital trustees on patient and staff microbiologic safety.

In many places where complying with good hygiene procedures is held in high esteem, good hygienic practices are demonstrated by nurses and other health care providers (Collins, 2010). Bed baths are sometimes included in these discussions; they have been replaced in many agencies by microwavable disposable bathing kits (Pipe et al., 2012) and other approaches and equipment. Nonetheless, bathing is still valued and promoted as part of patients' hygienic needs: "the patient's hygiene needs will be met on a consistent basis, through collaboration with nursing, to promote independence, and ensure a clean body" (Pipe et al., 2012, p. 232).

According to Holmes et al. (2006), the unclean side of nursing is rarely explored in scholarly literature. These scholars noted that nurses care for and yet implicitly retreat from abject or repulsive patients, such as homeless persons, rape or incest victims, burn victims, rapists, serial killers, pedophiles, or IV drug users. Nurses learn to reject their own sensibilities to maintain professionalism (Holmes et al., 2006) so that all patients, no matter how abject, receive care in close, personal contact. Responsibility for patient care is primary and supersedes nurses' fears of self-contamination.

Nurses deal with their contacts with profane materials with humor, complaining, fear, science, taken-for-grantedness, and tolerance. Bathing patients, whether using the traditional basin and washcloth or the microwavable disposable bathing kit, involves direct contact with the orifices of the human body and with invasive malodorous wounds. The genitals, anus, and mouth, along with the ears, eyes, and nostrils produce excreta and secretions that are profane. Contact with and control of these profane materials is accomplished by professional nurses and other nursing staff. In addition and among themselves, nurses acknowledge their rankings of potentially dangerous materials on the "hierarchy of yuck": sputum (and respiratory secretions) is more repugnant than feces; feces are more repellant than urine (Wolf, 2009, p. 183). Despite repugnance, nurses do not often verbalize or show their negative reactions in spite of their disgust, but occasionally do (Picco et al., 2010). They are "supposed to sublimate" (Holmes et al., 2006) their feelings. As frontline workers in health care, nurses are repulsed by some individuals and human products. In some way, the bath or bathing patients gradually minimizes feelings of repugnance and at the same time not only imposes controls for workplace order but also its patients.

SUMMARY

Douglas (1975) noted that, "relations with the sacred must be protected from the profane by interdictions. Relations with the sacred are always expressed through rituals of separation and demarcation and are reinforced with beliefs in the danger of crossing forbidden boundaries" (p. 49). Clean and dirty are kept separate using the bathing ritual and procedure. For example, patients who are soiled during vehicular accidents are bathed to facilitate careful assessment.

Nurses cross forbidden boundaries every day by giving intimate, personal care during bathing activities. As bathing takes place in privacy, the skill of performing this ritual is seldom witnessed by others. As hidden work, it may be taken for granted and underestimated in relation to what patients experience as they are cared for during bathing and the skill nurses demonstrate.

Patients are comforted when they are bathed. Whether bathing patients is a therapeutic nursing ritual and/or an occupational nursing ritual remains to be debated. What is evident is that the bathing ritual, if accepted as such, has been transformed by science, everyday practical techniques learned in the care of patients, technological innovations, and the progress of professional nursing over decades.

3

Postmortem Care:
The Last Nursing Care

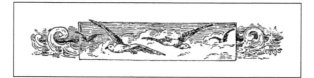

Nurses' work is closely associated with death. Even so, "Nursing care does not stop when a patient dies" (Quested & Rudge, 2003, p. 554). After patients are pronounced dead, nurses perform postmortem care, the after-death care given to their patients. Also called last offices, postmortem care is a nursing ritual. It is classified as direct nursing care in a British study on how nurses in intensive care used their time (Harrison & Nixon, 2002) and considered the final rite for the deceased (Hills & Albarran, 2010b). Consistent with other rituals, this care is directly associated with the practical work of nursing, and as such is a means to an end. Postmortem care also combines practices exemplifying the sacred and profane of nursing work.

In acute care agencies and long-term care facilities, nurses prepare the body for family viewing, the hospital morgue, and the funeral director (Quested & Rudge, 2003). Because of the pressure to admit other patients in recently vacated and cleaned beds in institutional settings, nurses frequently feel pressure to work rapidly to accomplish this after-death care. Simultaneously, they consider the needs of family members, not only to alert them to indicators of impending death if possible, but also to communicate skillfully with them after death occurs about typical activities to expect. Fear of infection can be addressed by requiring family and friends to use universal precautions and by avoiding disclosure of patients' privacy (Gelo, 1997).

There are many contexts of and antecedents to postmortem care. Patients' and family members' beliefs about death, family dynamics, individual preferences, cultural and faith traditions, agency policies and procedures, institutional, local, and federal laws, and national guidelines (Mellichamp, 2007; Wilson, Thompson-Hill, & Chaplin, 2010) provide structure to the event. Whether patients' deaths are anticipated, and if deaths are the result of violence, accidents, sudden deaths, brain death, vegetative states, failed cardiopulmonary resuscitation, mistakes (unusual circumstances), and acute or chronic illness also might frame the situation. In addition, health care providers' judgments about whether patients have "good" or "bad" deaths frame after-death care (Timmermans, 2005).

When life-sustaining treatment is no longer consistent with critically ill patients' preferences or the burden of treatment outweighs the benefit, withdrawal of various treatments influence after-death care. The threat of infectious materials may also be present, shaping nurses' performance using established policies and procedures. Likewise, public health concerns about infectious disease may call for strict protocols for handling the body, thus affecting care. Similar to other persons in contact with dead patients who suffered from infections, nursing staff in contact with potentially infected material need to follow principles of preventing disease transmission (Centers for Disease Control and Prevention, 1983, 2012).

In addition, the evolution of the hospice movement and more recent focus on palliative care have generated great interest in achieving quality of end-of-life care. When death is anticipated, care changes from curing the disease to caring and healing and helping patients emotionally, psychologically, and spiritually (Millner, Paskiewicz, & Kautz, 2009). Many strategies have addressed the need to eliminate depersonalized dying in health care institutions (Mellichamp, 2007; Walter, 2003) and denial of dying by society.

A multidisciplinary focus on the quality of dying for patients and the aftermath for family and friends has stimulated a look at how care for the dying is delivered and what care is provided for the bereaved. Nurses have consistently tried to accommodate the needs of family during the death watch and in viewing the deceased (Hadders, 2009). Nurses' clinical performance ranges from concentrating on a depersonalized view of the death based on procedure manual rules to providing their own empathetic style of clinical practice (Hadders, 2009) during postmortem care.

Fundamentals of nursing texts describe the procedure of postmortem care (Berman, Snyder, & McKinney, 2011), but students often do not have the opportunity to carry it out under the guidance of clinical nursing faculty. Consequently, many nurses are mentored by colleagues and actively participate in giving postmortem care with neophytes. It is also often performed as a group. In one hospital's palliative care unit in Norway, a "routines at the time of death" checklist has been created with the intent of protecting "relatives' potential need to participate at the time of death, to register their degree of participation when their loved one dies, and to raise nurses' awareness of the various aspects of postmortem care" (Hadders, 2009, p. 24). Family members may wish to participate in postmortem care (Quinlan, 1999).

In addition to nurses, there are many health care providers and support professionals who participate in the care of the dying and its aftermath. Chaplains (Walter, 2003), local clergy, physicians, social workers, law enforcement personnel, and crisis and bereavement counselors all may take part in events preceding and following death. Participants vary depending on the religious convictions of the person and family, the nature of the death, and the notoriety of the deceased. Interdisciplinary collaboration and active participation in improving patients' care help to assure that high-quality, end-of-life care is provided, including respect of last wishes. Holistic relief from suffering is accomplished through symptom management and caring practices for patients and families.

PREDICTING AND CARING FOR PATIENTS IN THE LAST HOURS OF LIFE: IMMEDIATE CONTEXT

According to Lawler (1991), nurses expect patients who are dying to gradually become more dependent and need more assistance as they get closer to death. Patients hand over their bodies, one function at a time, as nurses take over. The amount of control patients exert over their dying varies and depends on the degree of physical and cognitive deterioration. When nurses say they are "doing nothing" at this time, they are actually providing comfort care and emotional support. Doing nothing means that they no longer are intervening with care that is aimed at a cure (Lawler, 1991). "Dirty work" often predominates as patients' management of secretions and continence declines.

From the perspective of emerging nursing theory, outcome criteria for a peaceful end of life encompass not being in pain, the experience of comfort, the experience of dignity/respect, being at peace, and closeness to significant others/persons who care (Ruland & Moore, 1998). The standard consistent with this theory aims at achieving "peaceful and meaningful living in the time that remained for the patients and their significant others" (Ruland & Moore, 1998, p. 171). Nurses have consistently valued "good" or peaceful deaths (Wolf, 1986a) or what is termed *peaceful end of life*.

Preferred practices for care of the imminently dying were created to improve the quality of hospice and palliative care (Lynch & Dahlin, 2007). The National Framework and Preferred Practices for Palliative Care Quality Report detailed 38 practices. Six practices from Domain 7, Care of Imminently Dying Patients, are of concern for nursing. These are:

26: Recognize and document the transition to the active dying phase and communicate to the patient, family, and staff the expectation of imminent death.

27: Educate family in a timely manner regarding the signs and symptoms of imminent death in an age-appropriate, developmentally appropriate, and culturally appropriate manner.

28: As part of the ongoing care–planning process, routinely ascertain and document patient and family wishes about the care setting for site of death and fulfill patient and family preferences when possible.

29: Provide adequate dosage of analgesics and sedatives as appropriate to achieve patient comfort during the active dying phase and address concerns and fears about use of narcotics and of analgesics hastening death.

30: Treat the body after death with respect according to the cultural and religious practices of the family and in accordance with local law.

31: Facilitate effective grieving by implementing in a timely manner a bereavement care plan after the patient's death when the family remains the focus of care. (Lynch & Dahlin, 2007, p. 317)

Consistent with Ruland and Moore's (1998) theory and standard of care, nurses need to learn the indicators of impending death. Not only does this knowledge benefit patients' comfort, it also helps nurses predict the final hours for relatives and friends. Nurses manage frequently displayed symptoms, including pain, weakness, fatigue, immobility, lack of interest in eating and drinking, drowsiness, dyspnea, and delirium (Matzo, 2004). Peripheral cooling, peripheral and central cyanosis with skin mottling and discoloring, decreased urine output, loss of sphincter control, and decreased consciousness occur. Managing terminal delirium focuses on using sedation to bring patients close to their baseline mental status (Matzo, 2004). Near-death awareness, Cheyne–Stokes respirations, decreased secretion management, decreased stamina, and other signs signal imminent death (Lynch & Dahlin, 2007).

Signs of death are evident to experienced nurses. The patient does not respond to stimuli. Skin pallor accompanies vascular cessation of heartbeat and respirations. Initial muscle relaxation causes the patient's jaw to fall open and sphincters to release urine and stool. Pupils are fixed and dilated and the eyes do not blink. Patients' eyes are often open and sometimes this disturbs family members.

Physicians customarily pronounce or certify the death of patients. However, in some states and countries hospice nurses verify death. Verification of death may be governed by a policy such as one developed in the United Kingdom: no breath sounds by auscultation for 5 minutes and no palpable central pulse during that time. If during this time cardiac or respiratory activity returns spontaneously, another 5-minute observation period is warranted. After 5 minutes of asystole and apnea, absence of pupillary responses to light and absence of corneal reflexes are assessed along with motor response to supraorbital pressure. The time of death is then recorded (Academy of Medical Royal Colleges, 2008). In the United States, medical certification of death is described in a physicians' handbook (Centers for Disease Control and Prevention, 2003). When death is confirmed, patients' identification must be validated.

Physicians are advised to state that they have very bad news: that the patient has died (Frost & Wise, 2010). They share the reason for the death, briefly stating the cause, and if accurate, emphasize that the patient did not suffer. If the death was traumatic, a description of the effects of trauma is warranted. In the case of adverse or sentinel events (Frost & Wise, 2010), they should ask if relatives have questions and if they want to see the dead patient. Death certificates are prepared and used by families in preparation for funerals and estate business.

The transition from life to death may be initially difficult for inexperienced nurses to perceive. Perhaps the clinical indicators of death and lack of patient animation ultimately convince them. Clinical experience builds knowledge and recognition of the end of life. Direct nursing care activities provide nurses with an opportunity to not only understand death, but also to reflect on complex issues surrounding life and death and to understand their own perspectives.

TRADITIONS, BELIEFS, AND PROCEDURES

As a nursing ritual, postmortem care dramatically expresses nursing traditions. Rules of contact incorporate beliefs and dictate respect for the body and the way this body care is handled. Nurses are taught to protect the body of the deceased patient from onlookers and to care for it with respect.

Those who have cared for dying patients and witnessed their deaths have prepared bodies for funerals and burials for centuries (Jones, 1988). Nursing literature before and after the turn of the 19th century details after-death care performed by nurses (Burr, 1906; Tudor, 1890). An excerpt of an article on after-death care (Tudor, 1890) is included as Appendix A to this chapter. Florence Nightingale–era nurses and private-duty nurses in the early 20th century assumed this care from family members, and RNs, LPNs, and nursing assistants continued to give last offices or postmortem care to their patients throughout the 19th century to present day (Beattie, 2006; Jones, 1988; Pennington, 1978).

Professional nurses' concerns regarding caring for dying patients have persisted. Some responsibilities include: knowledge of the symptoms of death so that changes in patients' status are recognized; knowing how to care for the family of dying patients; answering dying patients' requests for spiritual advisors; saying prayers; calling for last rites; comforting dying patients by washing them, changing and straightening bed linen; obtaining desired food or drink; and medicating patients for pain with opium (Wolf, 1991a).

Much of postmortem care is performed in anticipation of viewing of patients' bodies by relatives and friends. Preparations include preparing the environment, preparing the body, and preparing the significant others to see their loved one. Privacy, cleanliness, order, consideration of other patients, body positioning and appearance, exposing face and hands, communicating sensitively, escorting relatives and friends to the bedside, allocating sufficient time for viewing, and assuring cultural, religious, or personal ceremonies or preferences require great attention (Higgins, 2008b; Hills & Albarran, 2010a).

How to care for a patient "once he has passed" (Myers, n.d.) is available to the public through web access and in health care agencies via procedure manuals (John Dempsey Hospital, 2012). Activities are specified through health care agency policy and procedure directives. Family members may wish to be present (Fallaize, 2007). Activities include: notification of hospital personnel, bathing the body or not bathing the body (depending on whether there are questions of criminal involvement, or if cultural or religious beliefs are present), covering wounds, replacing dentures, tying arms and ankles, removal of tubes versus nonremoval (depending on medical examiner involvement), tying on toe tags, placement of the shroud, disposition of jewelry and other possessions, transportation of the body to the morgue or other location, and completion and disposition of forms (i.e., death certificate). In the United Kingdom, oral hygiene is also performed (Hills & Albarran, 2010). Nurses need to ventilate the room and control offensive odors (Holden, 2006) and may use body bags to secure the body. They also organize the room in preparation for family viewing. In addition, the need to maintain dignity and respect for the deceased and gentle handling of an infant may be emphasized and explained. Directions were explicit in this example from nursing history:

> *Wash it [the body] piece by piece until all is washed. Keep the body cov-ered as much as possible, doing all as though the patient were still living. [C]lear away all soiled linen, nursing appliances, medicine bottles, etc. and make the room look as neat as possible....* (Burr, 1906, pp. 270–271)

Many of these activities in the care of the dead have been practiced for centu-ries (Jones, 1988, p. 27).

Shroud kits, clean linens, underpads, gauze dressings, a syringe to deflate a urinary catheter, and gloves, protective gowns, and face masks are assem-bled (Beattie, 2006). Concerns about infectious disease are addressed by uni-versal infection control precautions (Higgins, 2008). Shroud kits are available for adults, children, and extra-large individuals. An adult shroud kit typically contains:

- 54" × 108" waterproof, white, opaque linen finish plastic sheet
- Chin strap, pre-cut dual tape, 44" long
- One underpad
- Three ID tags with string ties
- Three 36" tape ties
- Two 60" tape ties
- Plastic bag to be used for personal effects

After patients are wrapped, hospital policies regulate moving patients off unit to provide refrigeration in the morgue to slow decomposition. When foren-sic evidence is required, postmortem care is modified and a chain of custody is added. Nurses have a role in collecting evidence according to protocols, including bullets, gunpowder and primer residues, clothing, and evidence required for victims of sexual assault (Snow & Bozeman, 2010).

Nurses have been responsive to family members' preferences sur-rounding the death of loved ones; many years ago their attention focused on religion-based practices. They have since gained more knowledge about the religious, cultural, or personal rites or routines of family and friends of dead patients (Hills & Albarran, 2010a, 2012; see Matzo, 2004, pp. 512–524). They gain some information about the world's major religions during educational programs offered in health care agencies and also ask family members about cultural preferences. Moreover, it is beneficial to have summaries of cultural practices available on agency computers or unit postings. In some cultures, the soul is disembodied and may depart following ritual ceremonies. Islamic practices may be performed by nurses to comfort family members, such as:

> [K]eep the body covered at all times; only professionals of the same gender should touch the body...encourage family member or friend to recite verses from the Quran...position the body toward Mecca...wash only excess blood, exudate, and excreta from the body... [ritual washing, the normal practice, is usually done by family members]. (Ott, Al-Junaibi, & Al-Khaduri, 2003, p. 229)

Another example shows that a nurse was sensitive to the cultural practices of a patient following a massive myocardial infarction and the eventual decision of a family to withdraw life support:

> I walked in the large room filled with many family members. I introduced myself and approached the patient, Earl. He lay there without movement or noise. The only sounds that echoed the crowded room were sniffles and the ventilator. As I repositioned...and suctioned his airway. I noticed a cloth on his chest, which had the earth, a bird, and fire sewn on it. I looked at his wife and asked her to describe the meaning of the cloth. She described it as a reincarnation of Earl. He was a healer in their tribe and this was a practice they performed when someone was going to pass over. Soon, I had to extubate him, remove tubes, and clean him up. I asked Earl's wife to explain to me what care I needed to take with the cloth while performing those tasks. She stated that I could remove it while taking care of him, but to place it back over his heart. I did just that, to preserve his dignity and spiritual beliefs. (Gallagher-Lepak & Kubsch, 2009, p. 179)

Some nursing units provide educational sessions to examine practices surrounding death and dying. An example of the contents of an educational program are the following topics: "communication skills in bereavement; understanding loss; reactions to bereavement; legal and professional aspects of death in hospital; attending to the practical issues of a patient who dies in hospital; cultural and spiritual diversity issues; providing support and information for the bereaved; and healthcare professionals' self-care" (McGuigan & Gilbert, 2009, p. 36). Intensive care units have incorporated underlying principles of grief and bereavement programs offered by hospice agencies into their plans of care and developed resource lists of formal bereavement programs in their communities to assist family members in need of interventions. They also place follow-up phone calls and attend 1-year anniversary memorial services in support of family and friends of deceased patients (Brennan, Prince-Paul, & Wiencek, 2011; Robert Wood Johnson Foundation, 2008).

Nurses' conduct during postmortem care shows that they respect patients' bodies and treat deceased patients like individuals. Often, they continue to talk to patients, telling them about what they are going to do

(Lawler, 1991; Wolf, 1986a). Their views on the body at this time are rooted in how they see death and what they believe happens at and after death (Lawler, 1991). The time between death and removal of the body can be experienced as a "breathing space" for involved staff (Speck, 1992).

Strange (2001) argued in favor of accepting the value of nursing rituals and analyzed what he called the *ward death ritual*. He described the details of postmortem care: washing and dressing the body in a shroud, and moving the body as a potential source of infection by conveying it in a disguised trolley to hide the death. He asserted that such actions free the bed for the next patient after it is washed with no taboo behavior evident about using the bed for the next patient. He noted that Lawler (1991) supported Douglas's (1975) position toward ritual; ritual defuses "the emotional distress generated by breaches of taboo" (Strange, 2001, p. 181). Nurses accomplish breaches of taboo, such as when they provide postmortem care, by virtue of the nursing role and its context in society whereby intimate touch becomes professional caring.

Nurses follow custom by keeping the deaths of patients in hospitals private. Contact with patients' bodies takes place in a private, personal place. Consequently, their concern denotes respect, but hiding the death does not necessarily protect patients and staff from knowledge of the demise. Timmermans (2005) argued that health care providers in hospitals and hospices have imposed greater control over the dying trajectory and continue to negotiate culturally appropriate deaths. His views provide another lens for nurses to examine postmortem care.

INITIATION TO POSTMORTEM CARE

Despite the fact that many people die in hospitals, nursing students seldom have the opportunity to give postmortem care in acute care settings. Their clinical experience is increasingly carried out in campus laboratories where they learn wound care, medication administration, and other procedures on simulated patients and models. The death of a patient may be the first time a student sees a dead person (Muir, 2002; Nursing Student, 2008). Most real nursing practice is gained day by day following graduation by reading procedure books and performing them alone with patients or by watching other, more experienced nurses demonstrate skills. In this way, the hidden work of nursing is learned (Biley, 2005). Learning the steps and using the equipment described in procedures are only a few aspects of postmortem care.

At first, touching the dead body may be difficult for students, especially if it is the first dead body contacted. Also being in contact with excreta and secretions that are potentially hazardous is threatening. Gloves and other protective clothing are used, and washing the body takes place procedurally, much like giving a bath.

Students may dread performing postmortem care for the first time and benefit from reflecting on the death of patients after the initial experience

(Keating, 2009; Mungall, 2008; Preston, 2011; Renouf, 2012). Experience helps. Performing postmortem care for a patient that a student previously cared for resulted in her appreciating the importance of dealing with the death of other patients and developing coping mechanisms (Mungall, 2008).

Staff nurses admit that little attention is paid to caring for patients after death in nursing education programs (Ward, 2010). The 10-step approach proposed by Renouf (2012 citing Kaye, 1996) for how to communicate with bereaved relatives helped a student overcome misgivings. She listed the following: preparation ensuring that the nurse is aware of all the facts before meeting the family; knowing how much the family already knows; assessing whether more information is wanted; informing the family that you are about to give them some bad news; allowing denial; providing explanations, if requested; listening to concerns; encouraging the expression of emotion; explaining what happens next; and being available should the family require help or support. Such strategies may allay students' fears that originate in aversion to the dead, cultural norms, anxiety about doing or saying the wrong thing, and other concerns.

Although being skilled at providing bereavement care to relatives and friends comes with living through it, students can be somewhat prepared by reviewing best practices. The FICA Spiritual History Tool (George Washington Institute for Spirituality and Health, n.d.) developed by physicians could help students address spiritual issues. F represents Faith and Belief; I, Importance; C, Community; and A, address in care. FICA cards include questions to ask and are available as pocket cards.

Contacting relatives or friends, directing them on where to go on coming to the health care institution, asking if they wish to be present during resuscitation, informing them about the death and allowing them to express their reaction, preparing the dead patient's body to look as peaceful as possible, allowing participation in postmortem care and time to talk, carefully disposing of the person's belongings, accommodating preferences that are cultural or religious, and mentioning bereavement groups are important functions (Kent & McDowell, 2004). Answering relatives' and friends' questions about the patient's death and situation requires honesty and respect for the patient's privacy, and giving advice supports them on practical matters. Once again, best practices help students prepare for this stressful and difficult task (Reid, McDowell, & Hoskins, 2011).

The benefits of performing postmortem care were described by Kwan (2002):

- Acknowledgment of the reality of death
- Fulfillment of caring responsibility by completing a traditional obligation
- A sense of completion
- Conveys messages of gratitude and respect
- Helps family go through the transition when they must cope with their relative's death

Nonetheless, giving postmortem care is stressful for nursing students and RNs alike. Nyatanga and de Vocht (2009) also emphasized the support needed by nurses and other health care professionals for their emotional well-being. They recommended having neophytes, whether students or practicing nurses, observe first and discuss the experience after the care is given. Even experienced nursing staff should debrief. The following reflection examines one nurse's evolution in the practice of last offices.

When I was a nursing student I encountered death about five times in three years. My paternal grandfather died. I vividly remember his viewing.

I remember washing the still warm bodies of four patients and recall thinking about the simultaneously subtle and stark differences between the living person and the dead person. Warmth was not solely associated with life. Dead people were still warm. They appeared very much like themselves. Yet the lack of movement of these people convinced me of their death, as did the progressive stiffness of their bodies.

Postmortem care was definitely a priority experience for nursing students. It included lowering the head of the patient's bed so he or she would not be flexed when rigor mortis occurred, washing the body, inserting the dentures, tying a toe tag on the great right toe, wrapping the body in the shroud, tying the shroud with cord at the neck, trunk, knees and ankles, and tagging the outside of the shroud. The patient's body also was covered with a sheet and the doors of other patients' rooms were closed on the way to the elevator. Many patients knew of the death anyway. The body was transported to the morgue by the morgue attendant.

As I look back, my teacher gave little advice about how to care for the grieving family. I comforted family members by my sympathetic, facial expressions. Words were simple because my discomfiture was great. "I'm sorry" was the best of my repertoire. The postmortem care procedure was definitely the emphasis. Faculty made certain I was "all right" emotionally as I performed the procedure.

Immediately after graduation, I worked in an intensive care unit. I saw many people die. My view of death was clearer because I worked against death. I "knew" these patients. I called doctors when I saw death coming. I prepared many patients for their families to view after death. Death was my adversary and my relief from strenuous work. I performed postmortem care for the families of patients so that the loved one could be seen on clean sheets, free of tubes and bodily secretions. I positioned their bodies in the bed so that the suggestion of suffering was removed and they were ready for the family visit.

So many of the relatives described the dead patient to be "at peace." I began gradually to agree with them, so that death became less of my enemy over time. Many of us, relatives, physicians, nurses, and nursing assistants, were glad that life had ended for many of these patients.

Death came to the ICU too often for my taste. In defense against death's frequency, I became overly organized in a functional or procedural way. Not only was I comfortable in predicting death, but death had become commonplace. How insensitive I had become.

It took time for me to recognize the impact of all of these deaths on me. I had seen too much death for my years or maturity. My feelings were numbed; I protected myself. My detachment had surpassed my concern.

Cortney Davis's poem (1997), "The Body Flute," provides other insights into the nursing experience (see Appendix B).

ARTISTIC PERFORMANCE

While it seems antithetical, nurses' artistic performance of postmortem care is apparent to uninitiated nurses and develops with experience shaped by repetitive physical demonstration and later reflection. Nurses mentor their colleagues, coaching them to accomplish after-death care as they communicate their respect for patients' bodies and transmit other values as well as knowledge about patients' and relatives' cultural and spiritual or religious traditions. Not only do they carry out the physical care of washing the body, dressing wounds, removing tubes, and other activities, they also consider the needs of the family and friends. At times, unit activities are extraordinarily eventful; consequently nurses might prepare the body and place it in the shroud, showing little evidence of the shroud's presence under the patient, so the family does not see it on visitation. "[T]he real challenge for healthcare professionals is developing artistic prowess to create such a peaceful, visually aesthetic appearance of the dead body" (Nyatanga & de Vocht, 2009, p. 1028). Done well, the patient appears clean and peaceful and the room is orderly with offensive odors managed.

There are unique accounts of inventive nursing in the context of postmortem care. Two other examples of postmortem care show nurses' respect for patients and families. An emergency nurse related how her colleagues gave postmortem care and arranged a private viewing of a young man's body in an emergency unit following his death from a narcotic overdose. His family and friends were welcomed and cared for. Another nurse shared a story from a Veterans Administration hospital regarding the death of a veteran. When the dead patient was transported to the morgue, his face was not covered. The body was covered with the American flag to signify service to the country. Another emergency unit nurse shared her support of the family of a dead child who had hidden in a box in the middle of a city street; the child was hit by a truck. The nurse decided that the parents should not view the child's body, cautioned them, and instead brought them to the emergency unit cubicle and showed them the child's hand with the rest of the remains covered. Violent death accompanied by external traumatic injury sometimes results in bodies becoming mutilated or horrible to look at, confirmation that death was not peaceful. This changes postmortem care. Nurses attempt to protect family and friends so that descriptions of patient suffering are hidden or minimized.

Research on Postmortem Care

Few studies were located on postmortem care. One investigator (Chapman, 1983), in studying cultural patterns of avoidance, described after-death care along with other rituals in hospitals. Others focused exclusively on postmortem care. Chapman's investigation is included in Table 3.1 along with others. Most studies selected employed qualitative methods.

POSTMORTEM CARE AS BODYWORK AND DIRTY AND CLEAN WORK: POLLUTION AND PURIFICATION

Early anthropologists linked ritual and death. Describing the tribes of Australia, Malinowski (1954) shared, "As soon as death has occurred, the body is washed, anointed and adorned, sometimes the bodily apertures are filled, the arms and legs tied together" (p. 48). The communal aspects of postmortem care are revealed on nursing units (Wolf, 1986a, 1988a) where nurses help each other through the experience. While rituals performed by family members and friends comfort them, the nursing ritual of postmortem care also helps comfort nurses by structuring difficult times (Pattison, 2007).

Douglas (1975) pointed out that cultural groups pay great attention to the symbolic demarcation and separation of the sacred and the profane. If rituals are not performed, dangerous consequences follow. Purifications, such as what postmortem care accomplishes, work in the space accomplished by this demarcation.

Deceased patients occupy a liminal place; they are on the threshold of life and death or life and afterlife, separated from the roles and statuses of the world (Driver, 1998). The everyday is temporarily suspended. Bodies are washed of the soil of death and indicators of suffering, positioned carefully, dressed in clean gowns, and placed on clean linens in straightened rooms. Dressings are changed; tubes are removed if permissible. Equipment is taken out and stored elsewhere. Nurses tidy up the patient and room and in so doing impose order on chaos as they purify patients.

Postmortem care is as potentially dangerous as any other "dirty" work that nurses do. Handling blood, excreta, stool, urine, and other bodily products is expected of nurses as part of the role. Contact with the dead is dangerous as well. Both contacts make nurses polluted or dirty by association. Not only does postmortem care performed by nurses and nursing staff take care of this needed function in health care settings, it symbolically continues the care of the patient after death and can be seen as a therapeutic nursing ritual (Wolf, 1986a). Practically, it demonstrates that nurses are often more familiar, and therefore closer, with patients than other health care providers, so it is not surprising that it is the domain of nursing.

The fact that postmortem care is the last body care patients receive distinguishes its activities. While this after-death care is often emotionally

TABLE 3.1
Reviewed Citations

Study/Article	Theoretical Basis for Study	Design; Question/Purpose; Sampling Frame/Size	Independent Variables (IV); Dependent Variables (DV)	Measurement of Variables (Name of Instrument, etc.)	Statistics Used to Answer Research Question	Level of Research (or Nonresearch Evidence) Results/Recommendations; Rating Strength of Evidence; Quality
Chapman (1983)	Weber's model of social conduct: Human action four ideal types: traditional action in which behavior is determined by action or habit; action that is purposely ions rational conduct in which there is a technical relation between means and ends; vertrational action whereby the means and ends of the action are not always empirically provable, although based on systematic set of beliefs or ideas; affective act carried out under the influence of some sort of emotive state	Qualitative, field study; ritual practices in nursing surrounding birth, death, status, and power; nonrational and rational ritual compared	Cultural patterns of avoidance: patient as a dying person and performance of last offices or laying out the corpse and washing it; clothed in white gown, labeled the body, wrapped in shroud; nurses wore gowns; group performance; ward curtains closed and body taken away on a mortuary trolley disguised by a sheet Hospital lifecycle rituals (rites of passage) also described, chiefly concerning dress, hats, and other objects, designating growth in professional maturity	Participant observations		Ritual has social and psychological meaning; ritual procedures are not only defense mechanisms against anxiety, but social acts that generate and convey meaning

| Wolf (1986) | Frame of reference: anthropological, sociological, and nursing literature | Qualitative, ethnography

What actions, words, and objects make up nursing rituals?

What are the types of nursing rituals demonstrated by professional nurses caring for adult patients?

What explicit or manifest meanings do these rituals have to nurses, patients, and their families, and to other hospital personnel?

What implicit or latent meanings are identified by the nurses, patients, and other hospital personnel, and by the investigator? | Context: medical nursing unit large urban hospital to study:

1. postmortem care
2. admission of patients to the hospital and discharge of patients from the hospital
3. medication administration
4. bathing, handling of excreta and secretions, caring for patients with infectious disease
5. change-of-shift report | Participant observation (fieldwork) and field notes, semistructured interviews, event analysis, document analysis | Therapeutic nursing ritual: the bath, bathing patients; postmortem care (context do not resuscitate dilemma); medication administration

Occupational nursing ritual: change-of-shift report

Patient ritual: admission to the hospital

Postmortem care was contextualized by the "resuscitate or do not resuscitate" dilemma. Postmortem care represented on a symbolic level a relinquishing of responsibility. Some nurses thought that the spirit of their patients still surrounded the dead patient's body. Nurses cleaned their patients' room and washed their bodies with an earnestness that reflected the need to purify the room and the body of the traces of suffering and the soil of death |

(continued)

73

TABLE 3.1
Reviewed Citations (continued)

Study/ Article	Theoretical Basis for Study	Design; Question/ Purpose; Sampling Frame/Size	Independent Variables (IV); Dependent Variables (DV)	Measurement of Variables (Name of Instrument, etc.)	Statistics Used to Answer Research Question	Level of Research (or Nonresearch Evidence) Results; Recommendations; Rating Strength of Evidence; Quality
		How do nursing rituals emerge in the context of postmortem care, medication administration, admission and discharge procedures, change-of-shift report, and the aseptic practices of nurses, including the bed bath and the care of infected patients? Informants: nurses, patients, family members, hospital personnel				
Wolf (1991b)	Frame of reference from articles from the nineteenth century, textbooks, hospital procedure manuals; postmortem care as a therapeutic nursing ritual	To investigate lived experiences of RNs in giving postmortem care in operating rooms to organ donors; registered nurses (N = 8)	Experience giving postmortem care in operating rooms to organ donors	Semistructured interviews		Clusters: organ procurement surgery of brain-dead patient associated with final death of patient; nurses have dual responsibilities—to donor and to recipient families; brain-dead patient transformed into organ donor; family's give is extraordinary: life from death; final death of donor is emotionally

74

				difficult for nurses; organ procurement surgery changes postmortem care; postmortem care: nurses' work; postmortem care: ritual and procedure
Eynan-Harvey (1996)	Historical, philosophical, religious themes on death; attitudes on death; attitudes toward death; funeral rites in context of culture; invisibility of death	Qualitative and quantitative; to describe nurses' postmortem care experiences and to determine the influence it exerts on their attitudes toward death; to relate variations in attitudes toward death to the type of hospital setting in which nurses work to the nurses' cultural backgrounds, and to offer recommendations; questionnaire completed by nurses (most RNs, few LPNs) ($N = 31$) Canadian ($n = 17$) and Israeli ($n = 15$) nurses; 7 nurses interviewed	Postmortem care experiences and their influences on attitudes toward death and variations of attitudes related to hospital setting and nurses' cultural backgrounds	Self-administered questionnaire (open- and close-ended items); in-depth interviews	Most nurses feared the dead body at the beginning of their clinical experience; nurses anxious and afraid of touching cold skin, deceased spirit, sudden spontaneous resurrection, and their inexperience caring for the dead. Fear more intense for Israeli nurses. Palliative care nurses had no reservations about touching dead body; medical nurses anxious and uneasy about it; most Israeli nurses expressed disgust and loathing. Conflict between showing respect to dead patient and time pressures; rewarding experience: ended prolonged suffering for patient. Patient transformed to body when shroud in place. Placing the patient in shroud most difficult task: dehumanizing and disrespectful. Postmortem care allowed nurses to accept death and complete grieving; achieve closure. Attitudes toward death influenced by many sources, chiefly by personal values.

(continued)

TABLE 3.1

Reviewed Citations (continued)

Study/Article	Theoretical Basis for Study	Design; Question/Purpose; Sampling Frame/Size	Independent Variables (IV); Dependent Variables (DV)	Measurement of Variables (Name of Instrument, etc.)	Statistics Used to Answer Research Question	Level of Research (or Nonresearch Evidence) Results/Recommendations; Rating Strength of Evidence; Quality
						Most support was informal and came from the unit. Death was conceptualized very differently among nurses, either the end or new beginning or transition; process of caring for the dying and personal values determined attitudes toward death and dying. Many nurses sensed existent of energy or spirit in room or around them as they cared for the body.
Hadders (2009)	Multiple discourses of death manifested and made real as much in procedure manual as in medical practice	To describe how and in what manner standardization and management of hospital death has evolved in a particular regional Norwegian hospital over the last decades; to describe the coordination of various enactments of death and the dead patient within late-modern Norwegian	Standardization and management of hospital death; coordination of enactments of death and dead patient	Tape-recorded semistructured interviews on specific death in the unit; document analysis of 24-hour medical record; participant observation of care of terminal and sedated ventilator patients		Some aspects of postmortem care need to be compulsory, and others are open to greater improvization; nurses inform relatives of the advance of death to discern participation and inform of activities; the term *corpse* is never used, most often, *dead patient*; nurses washing of the patient's body is done respectfully; nurses attempt to involve relatives in the death watch, postmortem care, and prepare the room for a viewing of the patient; nurses apply identity tag to wrist

	hospital practice; to argue that late-modern medical standardization of death leads to multidimensional medical practice; ICU nurses ($N = 28$); procedure manuals; 24-hour medical record sheet			Death in clinical setting is multiple affair, embedded in material, sociocultural, legal, ethical, aesthetic, and economic practice at collective and individual levels
Kwan (2002)	Rituals of transition (van Gennep, 1960)	Qualitative; to explore the feelings of family members who had participated in the performance of the last office for the deceased; bereaved family members ($N = 6$) from five families	Feelings during, reason for participating, meaning of participating in last office of deceased family member	Semistructured interviews: feelings during participation of last office; reason for participating in last office; meaning of participation for family members	Last office provides a sense of completion; is a continuation of the relationship between the deceased and family; conveys messages of gratitude and respect; helps fulfill each family's sense of responsibility to their loved one; important process to enhance the acknowledgment of reality of death as a humanistic approach, helps family go through important time of transition when they must cope with the fact that their relative is no longer alive

(continued)

TABLE 3.1
Reviewed Citations (continued)

Study/ Article	Theoretical Basis for Study	Design; Question/ Purpose; Sampling Frame/Size	Independent Variables (IV); Dependent Variables (DV)	Measurement of Variables (Name of Instrument, etc.)	Statistics Used to Answer Research Question	Level of Research (or Nonresearch Evidence) Results/ Recommendations; Rating Strength of Evidence; Quality
Questad and Rudge (2003)	Nursing procedure manuals include texts embedded with beliefs about nursing practices and how such practices meet societal influences and are shaped by them	Discursive analysis; excerpts of last offices in policy and procedure manuals; exploration of procedure manual and medical practice on how health personnel enact death and deal with the dead patient	Insights into social and cultural values that surround the dead, nursing practices and rituals involved in care of the dead, and the various medical and social categories assigned to the body throughout the manual excerpt	Critical analysis of use of language; questioning of actual language of procedure manual to determine the construction of the text to determine how things are represented in language in a specific context and at a specific time; text questioned about related nursing practice and performance (Foucault, 1972; Fairclough, 1992)		Language of last offices demonstrates the invisibility of death in Western cultures. Differing views of the body: the patient, deceased body and the case; people and dead bodies; textually mediated dead bodies. Nurses reproduce the social etiquette surrounding death. To move from alive to dead involves a transition during which the individual is reconfigured conceptually, physically, socially, and culturally through the care practices inflicted on the dead body. Nurses' view of a dead patient is a result of their beliefs and values.

	Conceptual framework	Design/Purpose	Phenomenon/Concepts	Sample	Methodology	Findings
Smith-Stoner and Hand (2012)	Conceptual framework: patient perspective, family perspective, organizational issues, and legal requirements	Descriptive phenomenology; to describe the phenomenon of postmortem care as expressed in written policies for health care facilities contained in the sample; to gain an in-depth understanding of the scope of care provided and any areas of controversy existing in postmortem care. What key terms describe the phenomenon of postmortem care expressed in the available sample of policies from acute care hospitals in California?	Phenomenon of postmortem care; scope of care, controversy	32 respondents/ policies from acute care hospitals	Descriptive phenomenology	Themes: inconsistent terminology; care of the patient's body; musts and shalls; focus on organizational order; support for family

problematic for nurses, more so if they had a relationship with the patient prior to his or her death, it is absolutely disquieting for those health care workers outside of nursing and the general public. Again people ask, "How can you stand to be a nurse?" Many recognize nurses' work as dirty or profane, most often verbally associating it with handling bedpans and stool. Not many know about nurses' responsibility to perform after-death care.

The management of the dead body has been relegated to nurses' work perhaps because it occupies a place on a continuum of the type of work women did over many centuries, that of caring for the sick and infirm of the society. The dirty work of nursing also parallels the clean work. Patients and nurses, by close personal association, are polluted or dirty. Both are cleaned: patients by nurses who wash them, living and dead, and nurses who practice strict personal and professional hygiene and infection control practices. Furthermore, the admonitions of Florence Nightingale and her disciples about personal cleanliness, moral conduct, and nursing as a vocation demonstrate nursing's beliefs, maintained today, about the dangers nurses encounter as well as the extraordinary access they have in the care of patients. This reinforces a view of nursing work as sacred and profane.

The dying and the deaths of patients are sacred events. Many nurses recognize this. They also acknowledge the spiritual, religious, cultural, and interpersonal concerns of patients before death and relatives and friends after death. "To walk with people upon such a journey is to tread on sacred ground" (Pulchaski, 2006, p. 128).

SUMMARY

Nurses often grieve differently than family members and friends when patients die (Gerow et al., 2010). They struggle to compartmentalize their grief in order to support those with close ties to patients. They learn early in their careers to create a protective curtain and are very influenced by positive role models about how to handle patient deaths. Compartmentalizing grief helps them to remain professional. This boundary also denies their feelings. They also are grateful for the prior relationships established with patients and families.

Nurses do not always know the patients to whom they give postmortem care. In the case of emergency unit nurses who care for patients in crisis, the relationship is short. Nonetheless, postmortem care is a therapeutic nursing ritual performed for patients and families. To some nurses, the situation is an opportunity to show respect to patients and their loved ones and to honor the sanctity surrounding the death of patients. Even though the patient has died, some nurses think that the spirit of the patient is still present in the room. The soil of death is removed if possible and attempts are made to minimize the evidence of suffering before death. Nurses see postmortem care as a final expression of caring.

APPENDIX A

Excerpt From Tudor (1890)

I would suggest that to carry out the wishes of the family is the first point, and without any pointed or painful questions, their feelings can easily be grasped.

I have yet to learn, why in every direction one is always told to wait two hours at least before washing. I can only say how far more easy is the work if done at once.

First get all you need in the room. Then if your patient has been carefully washed each day, there is no need to do more than wash the face, hands and lower regions, taking great care that nostrils and teeth are perfectly clean, also the finger nails. If the body needs to be washed, do so with the flannel and sponge used while in life; never use tow(el); it is harsh and rough and would greatly grieve any of the household who might be helping you. See that every part is clean...put on the clean dress...turn the body gently on one side and put on the clean under sheet...arrange the hair so that it looks perfectly natural...place the head in the position most usually seen, see that the eyes are shut, roll up a towel firmly...and place under the jaw...put the hands in a natural position, or over the chest...try not to let the person look dead. Burn at once anything that has been used and would be of no value. Dust the room and make everything perfectly tidy and pretty, leave the window open a few inches at the top. Get some white flowers and ferns and lay a few carelessly on the bed, one or towel in the hands. Flowers can be in glasses about the form as usual.

In infectious cases...lay the person straight and remove the upper covering except the sheet, folding them together to be burn(ed) or disinfected. Immediately have the shell ordered...the body can then be lifted in the sheets so as to avoid as much risk of infection as possible; the shell will of course be fastened down at once. It is a good plan to hold a small piece of camphor in the mouth while doing these duties.

APPENDIX B

The Body Flute

O my body! I dare not desert
the likes of you in other
men and women, nor
the likes of the parts of you
—Walt Whitman

Go on loving the flesh
after you die.
I close your eyes

bathe your bruised limbs
press down the edges of tape
sealing your dry wounds.

I walk with you to the morgue
and pillow your head
against the metal drawer. To me
this is your final resting place.
Your time with me
is the sum of your life.

I have met your husbands and wives
but I know who loved you most,
who owned the sum
of your visible parts.
The doctor and his theory
never owned you.

Nor did "medicine" or "hospital"
ever own you.
Couldn't you, didn't you
refuse tests, refuse to take your medicine?
But I am the nurse
of childhood's sounds in the night,
nurse of the washrag's sting
nurse of needle and sleep
nurse of lotion and hands on skin
nurse of sheets and nightmares
nurse of the flashlight beam at 3 a.m.

I know the privacy of vagina and rectum
I slip catheters into openings
I clean you like a mother does.
That which you allow no one,
you allow me.

Who sat with you that night?
Your doctor was asleep,
Your husband was driving in.
Your wife took a few things
home to wash, poor timing,
but she had been by your side for days.
Your kids? They could be anywhere,
even out with the vending machines
working out just how much
you did or didn't do for them.

You waited
until you were alone
with me. You trusted
that I could wait and not be
frightened away.
That I would not expect
anything of you—
not bravery or anger, now even
a good fight.

At death
You become wholly mine.
Your last glance, your last
sensation of touch,
your breath
I inhale, incorporating you
into memory.
Your body
silvery and still on the bed,
your lips fluttering into blue.
I pull your hand away from mine.
My other hand lingers, traces
your finger from the knucklebone
to the sheets
into which your body sinks,
my lips over yours,
my cheek near the blue
absence of your breath,
my hands closing
the silver of your eyelids.

     —Cortney Davis

Medication Errors and Medication Administration: Ritualistic Prevention

The Magic Number

3

The Magic Number

❦   ❦

Medication administration is only one multifaceted phase of the medication-use process. The complex issues associated with administering medications safely to patients across health care settings and in patients' homes are well known. Monthly tallies of medication errors, compared to other errors in acute care settings, continue to convince health care providers that a startling number of such errors take place. Many strategies and research studies have attempted to address this patient safety challenge. Yet, medication errors happen in spite of strenuous and persistent efforts aimed at prevention. Most medication errors take place in the administration phase (Bates et al., 1995).

Medication errors are variously defined. The National Coordinating Council for Medication Error Reporting and Prevention (NCC MERP) recommended the following definition for consistent use by health care providers (institutions), researchers, and software developers:

> *A medication error is any preventable event that may cause or lead to inappropriate medication use or patient harm while the medication is in the control of the health care professional, patient, or consumer. Such events may be related to professional practice, health care products, procedures, and systems, including prescribing; order communication; product labeling, packaging, and nomenclature; compounding; dispensing; distribution; administration; education; monitoring; and use.* (NCC MERP, 2012)

Across the United States and in many other countries, medication errors have attracted considerable attention owing to the workplace deaths and permanent injuries associated with mistakes involving drugs. These and other sentinel events (The Joint Commission, 2011) challenge the intellectual and strategic abilities of nurses, physicians, pharmacists, risk managers, patient safety officers, hospital administrators, and boards of trustee. All health care providers are implicated in the outcomes of medication errors as are the health care systems in which they work. Nurses work at the sharp end (Reason, 1995) of the medication use process and are positioned, and accept the responsibility, to catch errors before they reach patients (Folkmann & Rankin, 2012; Taxis & Barber, 2003). Patients and families trust nurses implicitly to act safely.

Health care errors connote personal and systems-based causation and call for explanations. Regrettably, patients, family members, friends of patients, and providers suffer the consequences. Nurses are devastated and recall errors for years afterward (Dewar, 2012; Treiber & Jones, 2010; Wolf, 1994). In addition, the costs of litigation tax health care agency budgets and health care providers' time when addressing claims.

Compared to individuals living at home who self-administer medications or give drugs to family members, friends, or employees, RNs administer more medications than others. They also make many drug administration errors (Carlton & Blegen, 2006). The knowledge, skills, and values needed for this task of nursing are substantial, especially in view of the plethora of medications (including high-alert drugs involved in sentinel events), their dosages, timing, side and toxic effects, accepted routes of administration, and need to monitor drug effectiveness (see Appendix A). Complicated by these factors are the work environments or environments of care in which nurses live and work. Nurse staffing issues (Dunn, 2003; Hanrahan, Kumar, & Aiken, 2010), units staffed by less-experienced nurses (Carlton & Blegen, 2006), higher acuity patients (Carlton & Blegen, 2006), multiple distractions, and interruptions (Nguyen, Connolly, & Wong, 2010) threaten patient safety. Transitions of care whereby patients move from one health care provider or setting to another also challenge medication safety (Flora, Parsons, & Slattum, 2011).

In addition, medication administration is inseparable from nurses' other work, thus making it only one part of many nursing care interventions. The cognitive load and cognitive shifts required by the differing care demands of patients challenge nurses' performance, and these factors along with multiple interruptions jeopardize patient safety (Potter et al., 2005). Medication administration calls for policies, procedures, routines, and even ritual protection from error. Medication errors require reporting and disclosure, as types of public confession, once administration errors have occurred.

TRADITIONS, BELIEFS, PRACTICES, AND DEFINITIONS

Medication administration has long been incorporated into the functions characteristic of the role of the nurse (Miller, 2011). Nurses have traditionally given medications; it is an everyday nursing activity and is linked to their professional identity. They are responsible to their patients and to each other to give medications safely.

Nurses share the serious trust of this function with physicians and pharmacists more than any other health care providers. Together, these providers subscribe to the ethical principles of doing good (beneficence) and avoiding harm (nonmaleficence). Medication administration demonstrates professional and personal commitment to the safety of patients. All believe in the therapeutic benefits of medications, based both on science and to a certain extent on magical thinking.

The science associated with the chemical effects of medications in the body convinces nurses, physicians, and pharmacists of their therapeutic worth. Yet, at the same time that they trust the effects of treatment, they also fear the possibility of what can go wrong. They have seen the adverse effects of medications administered incorrectly (Bates et al., 1995) and have committed errors themselves. The statement, "the medication is working" conveys the belief that the intended action of the drug has in fact happened.

The overt nature of medication administration shows in the repeated patient identification efforts as nurses prepare to administer medications. Also in evidence are technology and computerization in support of error reduction (Wolf, 2007): electronic health records (Jha et al., 2009; Scanlon, 2005), computerized physician ordering systems and clinical decision support systems (Johanna Briggs Institute, 2006), automatic medication dispensing devices (Mandrack et al., 2012), barcode technology for bedside scanning, carts, intravenous (IV) medication smart pumps (Hertzel & Sousa, 2009; Nicholas & Agius, 2005), and cordless phones. Additional equipment includes IV poles, packaged drugs themselves (blister packs, vials, suppositories, glass containers, IV bags, ointments, nebulizers, patient-controlled analgesia, etc.), related supplies (alcohol pledgets, syringes, needles, IV tubings, syringes, soufflé cups, measured medication cups, gloves, dressings, etc.), and storage of contaminated equipment available in unit cubicles and patient rooms. Medication administration records (MARs) and other elements of patient-related health care documents underscore the public nature of medication administration.

Drug administration requires nurses to demonstrate cognitive, psychomotor, and interpersonal skills as they use equipment and give medications to patients. They show patients, relatives, and friends how to administer drugs. They teach patients about the actions of medications and warn them about side effects. Not only do they learn how to give drugs via the different routes of administration, such as IV, intramuscular, subcutaneous, intradermal, inhaled, topical, vaginal, urethral, bladder, enteral (via gastrointestinal tube), oral (swallowed, sublingual), and via ear, nose, and eye, and so forth, they also teach patients the needed skills. Knowledge of anatomy and skill with how to manipulate the different forms in which drugs are manufactured is required.

Functions of Medications and Types of Medication Errors

Medications stabilize, treat, cure, comfort, diagnose, and prevent disease, modify signs, or reduce or eliminate symptoms. They also act prophylactically and as placebos (Blair, 1996). No matter the severity of the medication error (Hartwig, Denger, & Schneider, 1991; NCC MERP, 2001), there are consistent patterns across research findings on types of errors. Some types are: omission (missed dose), wrong time, improper dose, wrong dosage-form, wrong frequency, extra dose, known allergy, wrong choice of medication, unauthorized drug, wrong monitoring, wrong drug preparation, wrong administration technique, wrong infusion rate, deteriorated drug, and failure to follow protocol (Barker, Flynn, Pepper, Bates, & Mikeal, 2002; Bohomol, Ramos, & D'Onnocenzo, 2009; Gladstone, 1995; Johanna Briggs Institute, 2006). Common causes of medication errors include lack of knowledge of the drug (lack of awareness of medication interactions, incorrect dosages, incorrect mixing, and overly rapid infusions) and lack of information about the patient (inappropriate medication for that patient) (Bates et al., 1995).

Medication errors can be classified into four broad categories: knowledge-based errors; rule-based errors; action-based errors (slips); and memory-based errors (lapses) (Aronson, 2009; Reason, 1990). Knowledge-based errors are based on general, specific, or expert knowledge; rule-based errors misapply a good rule, fail to apply a good rule, or apply a bad rule. An action-based error is the performance of an action that was not intended (slips). Memory-based errors occur when something is forgotten (lapses) (Aronson, 2009; Reason, 1990, 2000).

INITIATION TO MEDICATION ADMINISTRATION

Nursing students pay immediate attention to the cognitive and manipulative skills required to administer medications correctly when they are enrolled in their first nursing courses. They learn about the delegated responsibility of drugs ordered by prescribers, including physicians and APNs. In beginning courses in clinical settings, they are challenged by the calculations necessary to determine correct dosages and IV drip rates for different drugs. They also learn families of drugs in pharmacology courses and soon recognize the extraordinarily explicit details and the implicit cognitive load required of nurses administering medications. Ideally, their learning flourishes in a supportive environment (Reid-Searl & Happell, 2012).

It is difficult for nursing students to obtain sufficient experience in medication administration when enrolled in nurse education programs (Wright, 2005). Clinical settings may not permit students to give medications and often clinical faculty start patient assignments for students with one or two patients to care for during each clinical day. The reality that students practice nursing on their faculty members' licenses is momentous for students and faculty alike. The number of patients assigned may not increase throughout the program, or only increase at program end during preceptored leadership experiences. That, coupled with the need to supervise students' "pouring" of medications, limits the actual number of experiences students actually have prior to graduation.

Nevertheless, school of nursing and health care institutional policies require that students are directly supervised during medication administration. Students are also supervised by RNs in clinical agencies (Reid-Searl & Happell, 2012) as staff who also have a significant stake in patient safety and in educating future colleagues.

While the cognitive load for nurses giving medications is not limited to calculating correct doses, the conceptualization of drug problems thwarts students' success and results in further limiting their experience with this skill (Wright, 2005). Mathematical skills include calculation and conceptualization abilities (Brady, Malone, & Fleming, 2009). The way drug calculation problems are taught related to set-up differs among clinical faculty, and this may confuse students. Many programs repeatedly mandate in the syllabi of clinical courses that students demonstrate correct calculations of drug problems before being permitted to administer medications. However, a perfect score is not required in some cases to obtain permission or clearance to administer drugs. Some nursing programs have standardized the way drug dose calculation is taught. Dimensional analysis as a critical thinking task is taught to foster correct solution of drug calculation problems. Dimensional analysis is a mathematical calculation method for converting units on a medication page to units of the drug ordered (Greenfield, Whelan, & Cohn, 2006).

In addition to teaching students the policies and procedures of medication administration and supervising them during administration, nursing faculty traditionally teach the *rights method* of administration, which requires the checking of seven "rights": right patient, medication, dosage, time, route, reason, and documentation. This approach has been expanded as far as the number of actions required, with many programs teaching students additional content on the medication use process, such as the breadth and complexity of systems specifically tied to safety (Harding & Petrick, 2008). However, faculty have continued to believe violating or failing to run through a rights method is associated with student medication errors. In spite of this prohibition or prevention strategy, they have questioned whether the rights method for medication administration should be used in isolation of other strategies needed to address safety threats in complex systems (Harding & Petrick, 2008).

RNs also make calculation errors and many have not used dimensional analysis for drug calculations. RNs gain most of their experience in administering medications during actual patient care episodes when they provide direct care. Their competencies build as they care for multiple patients and ongoing education is essential to skill and knowledge development. However, how intentional they or health care agencies are in developing expertise in the performance of medication administration is not widely known.

One approach to expert skill development is offered here, applied to a medication administration example. Expert performance of medication administration may be developed by identifying representative tasks of sufficient difficulty, for example managing IVs for critically ill patients. The learning activity might capture the essential activities associated with superior performance in this everyday nursing activity. Also needed are maps of the "thinking out loud" cognitive mechanisms that help nurses refine their representations even though they are already clinical experts when performing this task (Ericsson, Whyte, & Ward, 2007). Skill development is ongoing, required by new technology and medications, and ideally matched to patients' individualized needs.

In order to teach nurses so that superior performance results, deliberate practice activities need to be designed to improve specific aspects of their performance along with opportunities to reach performance goals with repetitions, immediate feedback, and time for replication and problem solving (Ericsson et al., 2007). Simulations like this are scarce. It is more likely that nurses use trial and error and rely on other colleagues as mentors to provide guidance on specific questions and to demonstrate clinical skills of medication administration. In addition, in-service education programs in health care institutions provide details about the technologies used in giving drugs, such as smart pumps, barcode medication administration, automated dispensing machines, and other new equipment or software.

ART OF MEDICATION ADMINISTRATION

Medication administration not only demands cognitive ability but psychomotor skill as well. The art of administering medications involves nurses' manipulation of equipment so that drugs are given to patients with the least pain and as efficiently as possible, such as when they give injections for analgesia or start IVs preliminary to administering medications via IV fluids. Another example is the dexterity required to administer eye drops. This is not only because of the eye's tendency to blink, but because of the volume capacity of the subjunctiva's lower fornix. It is necessary for nurses to wait 3 to 5 minutes between drops to the same eye, otherwise the therapeutic effect will be lost (Shaw, 2003).

Skilled interpersonal interactions also affect patients' responses to medications; effective communication can augment the efficacy of medications. The art and skill in nursing practice is used to convince patients to take medications. "Every offhand comment, body language, eye contact, tone and inflection of the voice, interpersonal style, subjective evaluation, intuition, anticipation and nurturing..." (Blair, 1996, p. 12) may influence patient outcomes. Providing guidance and information to parents of children with asthma requires ongoing interpersonal skill and demonstrations of inhaler administration by providers (Blaiss, 2007; Winkelstein et al., 2000). Likewise, teaching self-administration to elderly patients demands nurses' skill (Hayes, 2005). Customizing written and spoken instructions to correspond with older learners' need to match teaching sessions with previous, knowledge-based approaches may help them understand their medications and ultimately self-manage chronic illnesses. Fitting the message to the needs of different age groups demands creative approaches. Respecting patients' decisions about whether or not to take ordered medications is also essential.

Skill in medication administration is also exhibited by nurses when giving analgesics to patients in extreme pain, such as after total knee arthroplasty (Ginsberg, 2001) or when suffering from bone metastasis. Knowledge of pain medications, the effect of patient-controlled analgesia, changing from IV to oral routes of administration, management of side effects of opioid use, and so forth depend on nurses' knowledge and skill.

RESEARCH ON PREVENTING MEDICATION ERRORS

The studies included in Table 4.1 explore reasons medication errors occur and strategies to reduce or eliminate errors. They are only a sample of available literature when considering the dramatic increase in investigations on the medication use process.

MEDICATION ERRORS: RITUAL OBJECTS AS SYMBOLS AND RITUAL PROTECTION FROM ERROR

Administering medications involves giving objects (tablets, liquids, ointments, etc.) to patients that have the capacity to cure and heal. Because of this, medication administration operates as a therapeutic nursing ritual. The medications themselves symbolize being cured and healed, and whether these outcomes occur varies. This is particularly true when considering actions, side effects, and toxic effects of chemotherapeutic agents. Nonetheless, the actions demonstrated by giving medications not only represent the imperative to do good and avoid harm, but also a therapeutic intention.

Medicines can be equated with ritual objects. They symbolize the intention of nurses to improve patients' situations.

> The distinction between "medicine" as "drug" and "ritual symbol" is a very fine one, and it is not always possible to make it clearly. All things are felt to be charged with powers of various kinds, and it is the job both of the herbalist and of the ritual specialist to manipulate these for the benefit of society. (Turner, 1967, p. 332)

Turner and others recognize the power of medications, as described in studies of other societies, and also the power of those who prescribe, dispense, and administer them.

TABLE 4.1
Results: Reviewed Citations

Study/Article	Theoretical Basis for Study	Design; Question/ Purpose, Sampling Frame/Size	Independent Variables (IV); Dependent Variables (DV)	Measurement of Variables (Name of Instrument, etc.)	Statistics Used to Answer Research Question	Findings
Arndt (1994)	Medication administration, common nursing experience, everyday nursing activity and highly responsible task Nurses' personal identity closely linked with medication administration Human precariousness and learning from mistakes	Qualitative, interpretive research; nurses' experiences with medication error and the meaning the experience of having made a medication error has for a nurse; 14 nurses in group; 12 nurses in interviews; written self-reports from 6 nurses; 6 cases from professional conduct committee	What does it mean to a nurse when she or he discovers that a mistake has been made in the administration of medicine? What does it mean to the nurse who has made the mistake? What does it mean to nurses being involved in the situation; what decisions are made by the nurses concerned in such a situation? What is it like to make these decisions? What guides the decision-making process? What results does the experience have for the nurse who made such an error? What does it mean to personal and professional development? How are other nurses who are also involved in the situation affected?	Group discussions; unstructured interviews, written self-reports, documents from professional conduct committee proceedings		Themes: procedure of dealing with medication errors; role of medical staff; image of the nurse and of nursing, situation of student nurses, support in the situation of medication errors Key issues: subjection and power, identification and change; guilt and shame, reconciliation with human precariousness; learning from mistakes, teaching and learning ethics in nursing education Accepting or resisting reality of medication error is crucial for personal development Traumatic experience counteracted by colleague support Medication errors result in conflict that demand decisions Concern with what led to medication errors

(continued)

93

TABLE 4.1
Results: Reviewed Citations (continued)

Study/Article	Theoretical Basis for Study	Design; Question/ Purpose, Sampling Frame/Size	Independent Variables (IV); Dependent Variables (DV)	Measurement of Variables (Name of Instrument, etc.)	Statistics Used to Answer Research Question	Findings
Cheek and Gibson (1996)	Nursing as a social and practice-based activity Regulation of nursing occurs at organizational and state level Policies and procedures regulate nursing practice The way the nurse's role in medication administration is written about, spoken of, and thought about is a product of political, social, historical, and other structural influences. Theses discourses frame the way in which nurses themselves think about their role in medication administration	Qualitative, discourse analysis Medication administration and associated procedures that exist to govern the role of the nurse	Literature review: scientific/medical and legalistic frameworks in literature on the role of the nurse in relation to medications	Five rights; disciplinary measures; surveillance: drug regimens, double checks, incident reports, medication variance reports, quality assurance audits; perceptions of good (no error) and bad (makes medication error) nurses		The ritual of the five rights (rites) demonstrates that nurses are objects of and subject to policies and procedures; these normalizing technologies bring about conformity and may structure disciplinary procedures Nurses as docile and self-policing; reinforcement of control Nurses' acceptance of blame for medication errors reflects power relations in health care system Oppression can lead to resistance and change in medication administration procedures

Baker (1997)	Rules governing medication administration	Qualitative, descriptive ethnomethodology; nurses observed for 18 weeks	Nurses' definition or redefinition of medication error	Participant observation, field notes, formal interviews, shift reports, document analysis	Redefinition of error (if it's not my fault, it is not an error; if everyone knows, it is not an error; if you can put it right, it is not an error; if a patient has needs that are more urgent than the accurate administration of medication, it is not an error; a clerical error is not a medication error; if an irregularity is carried out to prevent something worse, it is not an error) In cases of real error, nurses' concern is protecting the patient Institutional rules (policies and procedures) used to make nurses' lives orderly
Wakefield, Wakefield, Uden-Holman, and Blegen (1998)	Reasons medication errors of nurses occur	Descriptive, predictive: to determine nurses' perceptions of reasons for medication administration error; nurses ($N = 1,384$) from acute care hospitals in Iowa	Categories of reasons medication errors occur	Survey, level of agreement (6-point Likert-type scale)	Descriptive statistics, e.g., highest mean interrupted while administering medications ($M = 4.34$) and doctor's orders not legible ($M = 4.3$); principal components factor analysis	Reasons nurses' medication errors occur: physician, systems, pharmacy, individual, and knowledge factors (factor analysis) Medication administration process is complex involving multiple interactions among professionals, patients, and health care environment

(continued)

TABLE 4.1
Results: Reviewed Citations (continued)

Study/Article	Theoretical Basis for Study	Design; Question/ Purpose, Sampling Frame/Size	Independent Variables (IV); Dependent Variables (DV)	Measurement of Variables (Name of Instrument, etc.)	Statistics Used to Answer Research Question	Findings
					with orthogonal rotation (physician, eigenvalue = 1.23), systems (eigenvalue = 1.72), pharmacy (eigenvalue = 1.01), individual (eigenvalue = 4.27), and knowledge (eigenvalue = 1.75) factors; subscale values; Cronbach's coefficient alpha, .65 to .71	
Taxis and Barber (2003)	Human error theory (Reason); active failures at the sharp end: Mistakes (failures at planning or problem-solving stage of task), slips/ lapses (failures at execution stage of	Qualitative, ethnography; to investigate causes in IV drug preparation and administration; 10 wards with 113 nurses observed; 483 IV drug preparations;	Causes of IV drug preparation and administration errors	Observation; interviews	Active failures in 256 (97%) of errors; 25 (10%) slips and lapses; 60 (23%) mistakes, 171 (67%) violations	Most drug preparations followed the same procedure Error-producing conditions: Handling technology, design of technology, communication, workload, patient-related factors, supervision

Study		Design/Sample	Purpose	Method	Findings
	task): violations (deliberate deviation from safe operating practices, recommendations or guidelines, but no intention of adverse consequences)	447 drug administrations; 265 errors			lacking, and other (trying to save disposable equipment Routine violations, "cutting corners"); violation-producing conditions, lack of knowledge and supervision; latent conditions, lack of appropriate training and design issues (e.g., ambiguous labeling, complex design of infusion equipment)
Eisenhauer, Hurley, and Dolan (2007)	Thinking processes of RNs	Qualitative, descriptive; to explicate nurses' reported thinking processes during the process of medication administration; RNs (N = 40)	Thinking processes during process of medication administration	Semistructured interviews; grand tour and other questions; audiotaping of nurses' thoughts during actual patient encounters before giving and immediately after giving medication	Category frequencies Safe administration of medications is more than technical mechanical process; nurses constantly vigilant Descriptive categories of nurses' thinking: communication; dose time; checking; assessment; evaluation; teaching; side effects; work around; anticipatory problem solving; drug administrations

(continued)

97

TABLE 4.1
Results: Reviewed Citations (continued)

Study/Article	*Theoretical Basis for Study*	*Design; Question/ Purpose, Sampling Frame/Size*	*Independent Variables (IV); Dependent Variables (DV)*	*Measurement of Variables (Name of Instrument, etc.)*	*Statistics Used to Answer Research Question*	*Findings*
Drach-Zahavy and Pud (2010)	Learning and knowledge management; effectiveness of learning mechanisms (integrated or nonintegrated) on medication administration errors	Cross-sectional, mixed methods; to identify and test the effectiveness of learning mechanisms applied by hospital wards as a means of limiting medication administration errors; cross-sectional with sequential mixed methods design; nurses ($N = 173$) working in 32 surgical and internal wards; 518 observations	Patchy learning will not be associated with decreasing medication administration errors; integrated learning mechanism will be negatively associated with medication administration errors; nonintegrated learning mechanisms will be positively associated with medication administration errors; supervisory learning will not be associated with medication administration errors	Observations to detect medication administration errors (structured observation sheet, nine prescribed steps in medication administration); interviews (iterative analysis)	Mean ratio of deviations from each of nine prescribed steps as a proportion of the number of occasions on which a specific type of error occurred in each ward, divided by the number of medication administration sequences observed in the ward; hierarchical regression to predict medication administration errors from control variables and patterns of learning mechanism	Integrated learning pattern linked to decreased medication administration errors Nonintegrated pattern of learning mechanisms associated with increased medication administration errors The supervisory and patchy patterns were not associated with medication administration errors

Folkmann and Rankin (2010)	Social organization of nurses' medication work	Qualitative institutional ethnography; to provide an overview of the way medication work is conceptualized in literature and to introduce cautionary note into enthusiasm with which nurses' medication work is being reformed	Focus on discrete aspects of nursing, medication practices, without separating that work from actual circumstances of nurses' unfolding shift of duty; dominant discursive frameworks through which nurses' medication work is interpreted	Search of literature: descriptive, theoretical, and empiric writing addressing nurses' medication work (medication administration and medication error); critical discourse analysis	Influence of biomedical model on medication work; legal discourse places emphasis on procedures and behaviors established to make medication administration error-free; nurses responsible to stop errors; rights methods (seven rights) and three-time check used to evaluate nursing practice; docile nurse produced. Controlling for error—a management focus; managerial strategies developed to prevent medication errors; technologies relied on to reduce the risk of human error and have impact on nursing care. Patient safety emphasized; adverse events monitored; system's analysis and culture of safety in development. Large amount of nurses' medication work not known or captured; need to understand what is happening in practice and how it is organized to happen the way it does

(continued)

TABLE 4.1
Results: Reviewed Citations (continued)

Study/Article	Theoretical Basis for Study	Design; Question/ Purpose, Sampling Frame/Size	Independent Variables (IV); Dependent Variables (DV)	Measurement of Variables (Name of Instrument, etc.)	Statistics Used to Answer Research Question	Findings
Johnson and Young (2011)	Time spent in medication administration activities, rate of medication errors related to administration, classification of errors, Aronson taxonomy as contextual, modal, psychological	Secondary analysis of incidents from Australian database of metropolitan hospital ($N = 2,132$); to revisit the classification of medication errors, using Aronson's classification system, to gain insights into how to support nurses in this major aspect of care	Classification into types of incidents (taxonomy) and harm and injury (taxonomy) into intersection of both taxonomies	Self-reported medication incidents, de-identified, in hospital database from July 2007 to June 2008	Types of errors ($n = 318$) with omission of doses highest (15%) 93% ($n = 295$) did not result in harm to patient	Types of errors: action based ($n = 73$); knowledge based ($n = 15$), memory based ($n = 9$), rule based ($n = 7$)
Jennings, Sandelowski, and Mark (2011)	Medication use process of nurses and the medication day of the nurse; turbulence in contemporary hospital environments	Qualitative, descriptive ethnography; the work of medication administration in context of other nurses' work	Temporal process of medication day capturing routines and activities that nurses repeat day after day	Field observations; formal interviews; document reviews; open coding		Nurses' medication day unfolded within temporal boundaries of shift; scheduled and unscheduled medications; time management as dominant strategy Demands: institutional policies; technical devices; patients; physical environment; medications themselves

100

Study	Framework	Design/Aim	Focus	Data collection	Findings
					Five rights of barcoding medication administration system did not fulfill all documentation requirements Demands of technical devices; patient demands; demands of physical environment Managing time: articulation work of putting together tasks, task sequences, task clusters' sequencing medication administration; clustering care with medication administration; multitasking during medication administration; individualized techniques for managing temporal load
Dickson and Flynn (2012)	Patient safety goal in the context of flawed systems; medication errors as failure within safety system rather than one of nurses' errors	Qualitative, grounded theory; to explore the nurses' clinical reason and actions critical to the interception of medication errors before they reach	Nurses' clinical reasoning regarding medications during administration process: thoughts and actions when nurses discovered that something is not quite right with medication	Interview (taped, transcribed): outline and open-ended questions approaches; field notes during one unrecorded	Patient safety is a serious concern of nurses; medication safety extends beyond five rights. Nurses interact with other team members, chiefly physicians and pharmacists

(continued)

TABLE 4.1
Results: Reviewed Citations (continued)

Study/Article	Theoretical Basis for Study	Design; Question/ Purpose, Sampling Frame/Size	Independent Variables (IV); Dependent Variables (DV)	Measurement of Variables (Name of Instrument, etc.)	Statistics Used to Answer Research Question	Findings
		the patient; purposive sample (*N* = 50) from medical–surgical units in 10 hospitals; theoretical sampling	and/or order; what are the thoughts and actions hospital nurses used to identify medication errors and prevent them from reaching their patients: What factors in the environment had an impact on the medication safety care practices identified by hospital nurses	interview; constant comparative analysis		Clinical reasoning: how nurses kept patient safe from medication errors; six medication safety practices (educating patients, taking everything into consideration, advocating for patients with pharmacy, coordinating care with physicians, conducting independent medication reconciliation, verifying with colleagues) Clinical reasoning process: managing clinical environment (coping with interruptions and distractions, interpreting physician orders, documenting "near misses," encouraging open communication between disciplines)

Magic Numbers

Just as health care providers act on the basis of scientific findings in support of therapeutic interventions, they also rely on magical thinking and magic numbers as protection from making medication errors. For example, one author listed strategies to reduce errors: There are "25 things you can do to save lives now" (Runy, 2005, p. 40), eight of which were associated with medications. Another time-honored use of numerology in the ritual of medication administration is the three-time check, proposed to help nurses avoid medication errors, which has roots in the late 19th and early 20th centuries and which continues into this century (Groff, 1896; Lohman, 1933).

The three-time, or triple, check is intended to prevent errors. The three-time check has changed as medication procedures have changed (Berman, Snyder, & McKinney, 2011). The focal points of actions have also varied greatly among settings, suggesting great inconsistency in the application of this guideline. For example, the first check consists of pulling or retrieving the medication from storage equipment such as a drawer in a cart or automated dispensing machine. The second check takes place when preparing the medication for administration. The third check occurs at the patient's bedside immediately before the medication is given. This example demonstrates inconsistencies that have developed regarding the three-time check. Consequently, the three-time check does not represent an absolute standard (Institute for Safe Medication Practices [ISMP], 2004), along with other magic numbers used in the prevention of health care errors. The following examples support this concern.

Triple check; it takes no extra time or effort. Next time you are drawing up an IV or IM medication, always check the vial three times:

1. Check before you open it
2. Check while you are drawing up the medication
3. Check after you have drawn up the drug (Terry, 2007)

You will *never* administer the wrong medication this way. Plenty of mistakes are made with wrong medications. So many drugs come in similar-looking vials, with same-colored caps, too (Terry 2007).

Or, check three things before administering medications:

1. MAR (medication administration record)
2. Doctor's orders
3. Pharmacy label (Center for Life Enrichment, 2009)

Or, check the bottle at least three times to ensure you have the:

1. Right person
2. Right medication
3. Right route (Center for Life Enrichment, 2009)

In addition to the three-time check, the *rights methods* have also evolved with additional functions added over time. The original five rights address the "five wrongs" of drug administration: wrong drug, wrong dose, wrong route, wrong patient, and wrong time (Benjamin, 2003). Examples of the *rights methods* follow.

Five rights of medication administration are:

1. Right patient
2. Right drug
3. Right time
4. Right dose
5. Right route (Blank et al., 2011; ISMP, 2004)

The seven rights of medication administration are:

1. Right drug
2. Right client (two identifiers)
3. Right dose
4. Right time
5. Right route
6. Right reason
7. Right documentation (Hudson, 2009; Wilson, 2006)

The eight rights of medication administration are:

1. Right patient
   - Check the name on the order and the patient
   - Use two identifiers
   - Ask patient to identify himself or herself
   - When available, use technology (e.g., barcode system)

2. Right medication
   - Check the medication label
   - Check the order

3. Right dose
   - Check the order
   - Confirm appropriateness of the dose using a current drug reference
   - If necessary, calculate the dose and have another nurse calculate the dose as well

4. Right route
   - Again, check the order and appropriateness of the route ordered
   - Confirm that the patient can take or receive the medication by the ordered route

5. Right time
   - Check the frequency of the ordered medication
   - Double-check that you are giving the ordered dose at the correct time
   - Confirm when the last dose was given

6. Right documentation
   - Document administration *after* giving the ordered medication
   - Chart the time, route, and any other specific information as necessary. For example, the site of an injection or any laboratory value or vital sign that needed to be checked before giving the drug.

7. Right reason
   - Confirm the rationale for the ordered medication. What is the patient's history? Why is he or she taking this medication?
   - Revisit the reasons for long-term medication use.

8. Right response
   - Make sure that the drug led to the desired effect. If an antihypertensive was given, has his or her blood pressure improved? Does the patient verbalize improvement in depression while on an antidepressant?
   - Be sure to document your monitoring of the patient and any other nursing interventions that are applicable (*Nursing 2012 Drug Handbook*, 2012)

The nine rights of IV medication administration are:

1. Right patient: confirm it is the right patient and check against ID
2. Right drug: confirm correctly prescribed and appropriate for the patient
3. Right route: is the IV route suitable (e.g., can the patient swallow orally)?
4. Right dose: is the dose correct for patient (e.g., weight, age)?
5. Right time: is the time too early or too late?
6. Right dilution/fluid compatibility: checked with local/manufacturer's guide
7. Right flow-rate, using PRR (right rate, release, return and reassess)/ local policy to ensure correct
8. Right monitoring: crucial to ensure patient response and safety
9. Right documentation: so that administration is recorded promptly and correctly (Crimlisk, Johnstone, & Sanchez, 2009; Lavery 2011)

The 10 rights of medication administration:

1. Right medication
2. Right dose

3. Right time
4. Right route
5. Right client
6. Right patient education
7. Right documentation
8. Right to refuse medication
9. Right assessment
10. Right evaluation (Academy of Medical-Surgical Nurses, n.d.; Berman et al., 2011)

The differences among the total functions or cognitive actions included in the above rights methods point to an issue with actual implementation. For example, the addition of barcode scanners and other technology to medication administration processes has helped nurses carry out rights methods at the bedside, adding steps or actions to the rights process (Rosenthal, 2004). That issue, combined with the variations in how the three-time check is applied, suggests a problem and demonstrates ritualistic behavior.

It is difficult to ascertain what and how both numeric checks have contributed to medication safety. Nonetheless, the three-time check and rights methods are procedural steps (Legare & Souza, 2012) or guidelines that are still used every day in many ways, and are performed as ritual action. The use of numbers is aimed at preventing errors, and thus protecting health care providers and patients from the consequences of such mistakes.

These guidelines are routinely taught in prelicensure nursing programs and have been practiced by nurses for decades. The three-time check and five rights have most likely dominated among efforts aimed at medication error reduction or elimination during drug administration. The details of the actions performed have been modified because of changes in medications and equipment and work patterns.

Numbers have long been connected to magic and ritual performance (Leuba, 1909; Murdock, et al., 1961). However, the span of nurses' immediate memory may be limited by the number of items, "usually somewhere in the neighborhood of seven" that humans are able to receive, process, and remember (Miller, 1956, p. 90). Nurses' recollection that they actually have used the *rights methods* (5 to 10 checks) when administering medications might be further compromised by interruptions as they shift their mental resources to address other patient concerns (Yoshino, 1993).

Nurses may find it difficult to remember one of the rights methods, possibly because of the large number of operations. All of these numeric protections, most often used repeatedly and silently, may represent magical thinking and imply protection from error. All of the numeric checks, from the three-time check to the rights methods, very likely have prevented errors; but how effective they have been is unknown. Furthermore, they can no longer stand alone nor have they been or should they be the only strategies used to increase medication safety.

Theories as Prevention and Protection From Error

Theories and models are being implemented by health care administrators and health care providers to prevent errors (Wolf, 2007). Failure mode and effects analysis (FMEA) is a theory of error prevention; it is used in attempts to prevent future errors. Applied to medication errors, a failure mode includes systems and processes that could lead to a drug error. A health care team might review a new IV pump prior to purchase and track the steps nurses might use to prepare and administer an IV medication. The team identifies failures in design, listing all the steps in the process that could fail and lead to an error. They diagram the process to be assessed and assess the risk priority, likelihood, and severity of failure. Ultimately, they redesign the process (Benjamin, 2003; Cohen, Senders, & Davis, 1994).

Health care professionals use root cause analysis (RCA) after an error occurs. RCA is also an error prevention theory to understand factors that underlie variations in performance, especially those that led to a sentinel event whereby a patient died or suffered permanent disability owing to a medication error. The team meets to analyze the root cause: what, how, and why something happened, with the intent of preventing future occurrences. Data are collected, causes are mapped, and recommendations are made to change practice.

Reason's (1990, 2000) human error theory, a cognitive theory, examines organizational failures that cause accidents to happen via workplace conditions that provoke erroneous actions of an individual or team or by creating deficiencies in systems' defenses. Three error types are specified: skill-based slips, rule-based mistakes, and knowledge-based mistakes. Reason (2000) looked at human error from a person approach and a system approach and described the Swiss cheese model of how defenses, barriers, and safeguards may be penetrated by an accident trajectory. Active failures (unsafe acts committed by people in direct contact with a patient or system) include slips, lapses, fumbles, mistakes, and procedural violations. Latent conditions are the "pathogens" within the system; they may "combine with active failures and local triggers to create an accident opportunity" (p. 769; Sanghera, Franklin, & Dhillon, 2007). These and other theories might serve to reduce or eliminate error. However, they are lenses and as frameworks provide some but not total protection from medication administration and other health care errors.

Confession, Disclosure, and Reporting

It is an absolute expectation in health care settings that nurses disclose and report medication errors to fellow health care providers, patients, and families.

This mandate has not necessarily been easy to carry out for nurses and other health care providers involved in errors. They are guilty at having made mistakes. Fatal errors or those that result in permanent injury to patients are particularly horrifying and devastating for nurses and other providers (Wolf, Serembus, & Youngblood, 2001).

Disclosure and reporting of errors can be compared to confession and are very public in nature (Wolf & Hughes, 2008). This is not only because of electronic reporting systems and health care records that document some details, but also by letters to patients and relatives and during face-to-face meetings with them. An apology can be "cleansing and venerating" (Crigger, 2004, p. 572). Furthermore, nurses and other health care professionals wish to make amends following errors (Wolf, 1994).

The terminology of error corresponds with that of sin: errors of commission (violate negative rules of action, as the sinner performs those actions that are forbidden) and omission (failure to perform positive rules of action or actions that must be carried out) (*Encyclopedia Judaica*, 1971; Wolf, 1989b). Medication errors are not sins or evil human acts; they are not intentional. However, the common use of this terminology suggests that such mistakes at work may be equated with sin and disclosure and reporting with confession.

Disclosure and reporting do not always result in forgiveness for the nurse by patients, family members, other providers, or himself or herself (Crigger & Meek, 2007). Healing may be difficult to achieve. Whether reconciliation and absolution occur following a genuine apology (Taft, 2005) and if reparations are made are not clear as well.

SUMMARY

Medication administration incorporates ritual activity. Perhaps the associated ritual action fills in where scientific rationale fails. As a shared function in health care, medication use processes and drug administration involve many providers and complex activities. Consequently, errors involving drugs can and do happen simply because people and systems are fallible.

The evolution of the culture in health care agencies from blame to safety to that of a just culture has been influenced by many factors, including research and consensus about the main attributions of drug error: persons and systems. Hesitancy or fear of reporting near misses or actual errors is a barrier to safety (Maricle, Whitehead, & Rhodes, 2007). Thankfully, the shift of responsibility has moved away from individuals toward systems (Carlton & Blegen, 2007). Health care administrators are now convinced that to accomplish increased reporting of near misses and actual medication errors, staff fears about retribution and blame need to be eliminated. However, administrators are also aware of the reality that some direct care providers violate rules and thus place patients and agencies in great jeopardy.

Systems improvements continue to be carried out as errors are scrutinized and causes are reduced and eliminated. However, staff education and training are needed (Tissot et al., 1999) throughout each year to help nurses and other health care providers stay current on the complex knowledge and skills fundamental to medication administration.

More attention needs to be paid to analyzing the many examples of the three-time check and the rights methods. As broadly stated goals of safety in medication administration, they work to achieve safety. However, they do not stand alone (ISMP, 2007). Combining the rights methods with routines, rules, procedures, guidelines, and error theories may help nurses feel a sense of protection from making drug errors. All of these protections are insufficient for eliminating medication errors. Implementing theories of error prevention provide much promise for this outcome.

Team learning needs to increase (Drach-Zahavy & Pud, 2010) so that nurses, physicians, and pharmacists appreciate the challenges of new medications and technologies. Intimidation needs to decrease and systems improvements need to increase.

Nurses' work throughout the activities of the medication use process is complex. Changes, while ultimately error reducing, have an impact on nurses' vulnerability to making errors. Nurses at the sharp end must be more intensely involved in planning for the introduction of technologies that aim to reduce error.

APPENDIX A

Affirmation
Respecting the Selection of Alternative 4
for Providing Sentinel Event–Related Information to The Joint Commission

On behalf of [organization name] _____,
I hereby affirm that the following specific legal considerations pertaining to the relevant statutes, existing privileges, and case law have been reviewed as the basis for determining the most appropriate alternative available to [organization name] _____ for sharing sentinel event-related information with The Joint Commission. Specifically, the organization has:

- Identified and reviewed peer review and/or relevant statutes;
- Examined whether its peer review or similar committee, which has prepared or will prepare the root cause analysis and Improvement Plan in response to a sentinel event as defined by The Joint Commission (collectively "sentinel event response information"), is protected under its state's peer review and/or related state statutes;
- Examined whether sentinel event response information is protected from disclosure under its state's peer review and/or related state statutes as proceedings and/or records of a peer review or similar committee;
- Examined whether sentinel event response information is protected from disclosure under its state's peer review and/or related state statutes as proceedings and/or records of The Joint Commission;
- Examined whether its state's peer review and/or related state statutes permit disclosure of sentinel event response information to the Joint Commission without waiving the protections afforded to peer review materials;
- Examined whether case law in the state addresses any of the specific issues described above;
- Examined whether any risk of waiving legal protections for sentinel event response information can be eliminated or substantially reduced by appointing or designating The Joint Commission (by contract or other means) as a member of, consultant to, or participant in the activities of, its peer review or similar committee;
- Examined whether sentinel event response information is protected from disclosure under any common law privilege or principle in its state such as (i) the peer review privilege; (ii) the self-critical analysis privilege; (iii) the work product doctrine; or (iv) the attorney–client privilege;

I further affirm that on behalf of [organization name] _____ I

1. have determined that a root cause analysis which, to the best of my knowledge and belief, is thorough and credible as those terms are defined by The Joint Commission, has been completed by this organization for the event under review by The Joint Commission;

2. have considered the Sentinel Event Policy and Alternative 1, Alternative 2, and Alternative 3 (as referenced in the transmittal letter) for providing root cause analysis and other sentinel event-related information to the Joint Commission and;

3. have concluded that use of any of these other alternatives may increase the risk of waiving existing confidentiality protections for this information.

_____   _____

CEO   Date

Source: The Joint Commission (2009, April 1).

II

Rituals of Socialization

Section II examines rituals of socialization and integration into the professional nursing role. Change-of-shift reports are discussed from the viewpoints of background, traditions, research, and symbology. As a nursing ritual of socialization, it carries out the transmission of beliefs, norms, and values and communicates crucial information concerning patients from nurses responsible for their care.

Nursing ceremonies similarly transmit aspects of the culture of nursing. Ceremonies for nursing students are built on nursing traditions. Those traditions in celebration of nurses' work are tangible recognition of nursing excellence. They are performed by health care organizations and professional nursing organizations.

5

Change-of-Shift Report:
Rite of Passage for
Professional Nurses

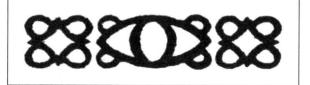

The change-of-shift report, intershift report, shift report, end-of-shift report, or handover, represent an opportunity for nurses to exchange vitally important and necessary information about patients under their care. The change-of-shift report assures continuity of care, signifies a change in the nurses providing care, and contributes to the quality of patient care (McCloughen, O'Brien, Gillies, & McSherry, 2008). Shift report exemplifies the continuous coverage of patients in health care agencies providing 24-hour ervices.

In contrast, the term *handoff* is often used in the United States to characterize the transfer of responsibility among health care providers at random times during the daily cycle. These transitions of care take place frequently; for example, when patients are moved from an emergency unit to an inpatient hospital unit. Handoffs are typically shorter than change-of-shift reports. Both shift report and handoff exemplify the process of transferring care and accountability for a patient from one health care professional to another (Blouin, 2011) in a concentrated process. Both change-of-shift reports and handoffs represent nursing transitions of care (MacDavitt, Cieplinski, & Walker, 2011).

The importance of the accuracy, completeness, and timeliness of information shared during a shift report is undeniable. It is a foundation for the next shift's provision of patient care; congruence of shift report information with patient status is essential (Strople & Ottani, 2006). Change-of-shift report, intershift report, shift report, or handover are used interchangeably to examine this condensed, communication episode in nursing practice. It is an occupational nursing ritual whereby nurses learn what it means to be a nurse (Wolf, 1986a, 1988a) and signifies a time when nurses are in temporary possession of the health and well-being of a group of patients.

The purpose of a shift report is clear to nursing staff and is predominantly retrospective, focusing on patient events during the previous shift (McCloughen et al., 2008). Shift reports also focus on predicted and pending tasks (Matic, Davidson, & Salamonson, 2010). A change-of-shift report is conducted among nurses in face-to-face encounters in private staff rooms, at patients' bedsides, or immediately outside patients' hospital, long-term care facility, hospice, or rehabilitation institution rooms during walking rounds. Sometimes, a shift report is presented in writing or is audiotaped for the on-coming shift's nurses.

A shift report is composed of three phases: prehandover; intershift meeting provided through an actual report; and posthandover, or the taking over of nursing care by the new shift (Kerr, 2002). Reporting progresses in an orderly fashion, yet interruptions are common (Banks, 1999; Evans, Grunawalt, McClish, Wood, & Friese, 2012). The time taken to accomplish this communication varies as does the pace of the delivery. The speed of medical-surgical, intensive care, emergency, long-term care, and rehabilitation unit reports varies greatly.

Attendance at a shift report by charge nurses and direct care nursing staff is mandatory for off-going and on-coming nurses. Delays in beginning the narrative result while staff wait for the presence of key nurses. As soon as the group assembles, a shift report begins.

Time spent in a shift report decreases when nurses change practice from taped or verbal reports to bedside reports. This outcome is explained when various types of patient-oriented documents that focus the presentation consequently structure the narrative (Athwal, Fields, & Wagnell, 2009). Also contributing to shortened time for a report is nurses' actions when attending to patient questions and needs during the transition period. Reports may be structured by printed, problem-oriented report forms, electronic, computerized handover tools (Matic et al., 2010), change-of-shift report sheets (Mosher & Bontomasi, 1996), care plans, and by nurses' personally created documents on scraps of paper or small notebooks carried in nurses' pockets throughout the shift (Hardey, Payne, & Coleman, 2000). An example of a computer-based change-of-shift report template in Microsoft Excel was created to standardize and increase the consistency of patient information (Nelson & Massey, 2010). Nurses updated critical data during the shift, then printed and presented it to on-coming nurses. A template served as the basis and a guide for the shift report.

Nursing staff have created transitions-of-care reports to standardize intershift communication (MacDavitt et al., 2011). The development of electronic health records for structuring a shift report supplements the traditional nursing practice of a shift report. Electronic health records hold great promise for increasing patient safety especially when applied to nurse-to-nurse communication. The creation of an integrated shift report with data from multidisciplinary records is aimed at fostering patent safety by including essential details on patients (Strople & Ottani, 2006), and is projected to formalize reports.

Consistent with shorter handoffs or staff huddles, a change-of-shift report provides an opportunity to alert colleagues to patient difficulties, intuitions about patients' likelihood of "going bad," health care errors, and unfinished work that needs attention. Details of new or unfamiliar medications, equipment, or care processes are also taught (Griffin, 2010). Nurses use the time together to express personal feelings and concerns of patients and families (Scovell, 2010). This highly complex communication event serves a multiplicity of practical functions (Kerr, 2002).

Nurses' interactions during shift report may not always be supportive (Blouin, 2011), so that a shift report's seriousness about patient issues may be complicated by sensitive, difficult, nurse-to-nurse relationships. Nurses may complain about not receiving adequate information to provide effective patient care (Athwal et al., 2009), or incomplete work was left for the next shift to finish (Sims, 2003). Nurse-to-nurse conflicts where criticism predominates and a "they versus us" approach that characterizes power issues toward physicians are counterproductive and require change. Such conflicts and problematic communications during a report could constitute safety threats; these patterns of communication need to be eliminated (Anderson & Mangino, 2006; Jukkala, James, Autrey, & Azuero, 2012). A shift report ideally functions to communicate information consistently to promote patient safety and best practices (Caruso, 2007).

Shift reports have also been criticized as unproductive and time consuming (Cleary, Walter, & Horsfall, 2009). Interruptions are common (Banks, 1999; Gagneaux & Shaver, 1977). Issues with traditional verbal shift reports include length, excessive overtime, inadequate reports, variable details about patients, and inability to meet patients' needs (Baldwin & McGinnis, 1994; McCloughen et al., 2008). Lack of a specific structure for a report can cause inconsistency and errors in report details. Patients and relatives can be stereotyped as being difficult (Wolf, 2010), and different nurses may focus on details they consider important and thus miss essential information. Some health care organizations have created standardized procedures to decrease variance and improve satisfaction and quality (Cleary et al., 2009; MacDavitt et al., 2011; Sims, 2003). Similar to other electronic health records (While & Dewsbury, 2011), information and communication technology developed for shift reports could result in improved information exchange.

Problematic shift reports that did not describe patients' situations completely have resulted in litigation. An example resulted in a sentinel event associated with deficiencies in the shift report. Failure to report suicidal ideation of a patient did not alert the on-coming nurse. The patient committed suicide. Such a serious outcome not only confirms the importance of intershift report information, but the necessity of using mechanisms to improve it (Strople & Ottani, 2006).

An intershift report also promotes team building (Speas, 2006). Strategies to promote team building have been suggested. They include signing a teamwork expectation contract; developing guidelines to include information in a shift report; exploring different ways staff communicate; promoting staff listening skills; encouraging staff members' participation in education of their peers; having a no-tolerance policy for rumors and backstabbing behaviors; and starting a reward program for team building (Speas, 2006).

The importance of effective communication among health care providers is dramatized by current patient safety initiatives. In 2005, the Joint Commission on Accreditation of Healthcare Organizations reported that the leading root cause of sentinel events was communication (Scalise, 2006). The Joint Commission continues to promote improved communication among health care team members as a major strategy to increase safety. Changes in shift reports addressing improvements in their context and content will most likely reduce risk factors and improve patient safety.

TRADITIONS, BELIEFS, AND DEFINITIONS

An antecedent of the change-of-shift report emerged as a precursor, located during a search for evidence of nursing rituals in pre-20th-century nursing journals published in the United States. The following description appeared in *The Nightingale* (1889) from Babies' Hospital of the City of New York. **The reprinted version duplicates the original format, punctuation, and spelling.**

Points for Daily Reports

Temperature—If pack, how long applied and how frequently changed. If Sponging, how often and how long at a time. Note effect of either. Note condition of child when temperature high, i.e.: whether surface warm or cold, or changed in color, child quiet or restless. If temperature subnormal, extremities cold, note effect of hot bags.

Sleep—Amount during day or night, if quiet or restles[s].

Awake—Quiet or restles[s]. Rolling head, staring, stiffness of body or limbs.

Pulse—Number and quality.

Vomiting—If nausea. If projectile. Odor of matter vomited.

Food—Amount in 24 hours. Appetite.

Sweating—Warm or clammy.

Urine—Color if any. Estimated amount in 24 hours.

Stools—Number and character. Acidity, if any.

Cough—Frequency and duration of paroxysms.

Eruption—Report at once.

Note New symptoms. All foods and medicines are to be tasted by nurse before giving to child. (Babies Hospital of the City of New York, 1889, p. 3)

The change-of-shift report accomplishes different functions. Patient information is provided, nursing staff are taught, errors are reduced or eliminated, and unit business is addressed (Cleary et al., 2009). Handover functions include providing information (patient reports, patient updates, family problems), being social (supportive, socializing), organizing the upcoming shift (planning the shift and patient-to-nurse allocation), and educating the nursing staff (teaching, socialization) (Wolf, 1986a, 1988a). As a nurse-to-nurse communication event, it is conducted in a group meeting or in a one-to-one dyad.

Hansten and Washburn (1999) summarized change-of-shift report functions. Explicit functions included "acknowledging signs and symptoms of disease; reporting on lab tests, specimen collection, diagnostic tests; ongoing discussion of patient's short-term (shift) outcomes as well as long-term (discharge or posttransfer) outcomes; feedback; education or training;

planning/department problem solving" (p. 26). Explicit functions listed were: "complaining in a safe forum; expressing humor (to help manage crises, stress, sorrow); initiating new graduates into the role of RN; warnings and acknowledgment of errors; war stories; monitoring of nursing care; completing unfinished business and passing on responsibility" (p. 26).

Nurses use terminology to describe physiologic, sociologic, cultural, and personal patient information. Because organization-specific terminology and nursing jargon is used during report, nurses exclude others from shift report interchanges. Language mixes formal and informal jargon (Strange, 1996) and has been described as cryptic (Payne, Hardey, & Coleman, 2000). Patients' social history may not be described in the case of older patients represented as "biomedically defined bodies" (Payne et al., 2000, p. 281). Less formal speech precedes the more factual communication. The special in-group language of a shift report is colloquial, scientific, technical, descriptive, and abstract with new nurses gradually learning it and seasoned nurses translating it (Ekman & Segesten, 1995; Wolf, 1989c).

Medical terminology is used during a shift report when describing diagnosis and treatment, and passive voice is used as well (Payne et al., 2000). Technology is described with language describing basic and complex nursing care. Euphemisms portray taboo topics, such as "going out" and "coded" (Wolf, 1989c). Abbreviations (such as OOB [out of bed]) and acronyms (such as CABG [coronary artery bypass graft]) help shorten the time taken with such communications. Hospitals publish lists of abbreviations and acronyms as part of attempts to standardize verbal and written communications. The following examples demonstrate those selections:

ABI, ankle brachial index
bs, bowel sounds
BS, blood sugar
BRP, bathroom privileges
C/O, complains of
CPAP, continuous positive airway pressure
DOE, dyspnea on exertion
ETT, endotracheal tube
FHS, fetal heart sounds
G-6-P-D, glucose-6-phosphate dehydrogenase
HEENT, head, ears, eyes, nose, and throat
HOB, head of bed
I & O, intake and output
L & W, living and well
MRI, magnetic resonance imaging
N/A, not applicable
OBS, organic brain syndrome
P & A, percussion and auscultation
quad, quadriplegia

RICE, rest, ice, compression, elevation
SH, social history
TURP, transurethral resection of prostate
URQ, upper right quadrant
VDRL, venereal disease research laboratory
WNL, within normal limits
XRT, x-ray therapy
yo, years old
Zn, Zinc

Nurses also use slang associated with bodily functions (such as fungy) and patient behavior (such as frequent flyer).

Language is terse and prepositions are used in awkward ways. Terse expressions are used to explain elaborate concepts (Wolf, 1989c). In a study on an adolescent residential psychiatric unit, the amount of jargon provided holistic assessments of patient behavior and mental state. Nurses "drew on collective experience with previous cases as a shorthand way of encapsulating information and care planning…this shared referentiality was a marker of insider identity which afforded a measure of professional pride and solidarity among team members" (Yonge, 2008, p. 48). In this study, irreverent descriptors and bad language were used and may have contributed to positive group morale. Language and types of information are somewhat similar across agencies, but differ according to specialty (Lamond, 2000), services provided, and product lines.

The content of shift reports is comprised of a great amount of information. Content is repeated often during change-of-shift reports and is characteristically redundant (Carrington, 2012). Some points of information are given in a specific order at the beginning of a shift report. (Lamond, 2000; Payne et al., 2000). General information, physical information, physical measures, functional, psychologic, social, family, nursing interventions, medical treatment, global judgments, and management issues are shared (Lamond, 2000). Most frequently noted information includes admission diagnosis, reason for admissions, significant findings, procedures, treatments, PRN medication, physical assessments, laboratory data/scheduled tests, respiratory care, and change in condition (Banks, 1999). Global statements are made about patients' physiologic status and patients are labeled, occasionally using stereotypes (Strople & Ottari, 2006).

When nurses report a decrease in hemoglobin and hematocrit, low blood pressure, and fever and pain during a shift report, they may be identifying precursors of common complications: shock, bleeding, pneumonia, deep vein thrombosis, or sepsis. Such complications could lead to failure to rescue patients and death (Carrington, 2012). Nurses' responsibility to anticipate possible complications may be shared during a change-of-shift report. While these results were generated on nurses' descriptions of clinical events, this investigation (Carrington, 2012) emphasized the importance of nurse-to-nurse communication during change-of-shift reports.

Details are always important during a shift report, such as whether patients' status is changing suggesting complications, or when they have DNR orders and living wills stipulating no cardiopulmonary resuscitation. Performing resuscitation without patient consent could be considered battery (Austin, 1996). Facts are commonly exchanged and are often critically important.

Shift report takes place in unit offices, nurses' lounges or break rooms, nurses' stations, at patients' bedsides, chair sides, or in the hall. Nurses monitor the volume of their speech, and avoid "talking over" patients when bedside rounds are conducted. Nurses often deliberately involve patients (Scovell, 2010), yet it is important that as the amount and complexity of information and treatment options often require privacy owing to concerns with confidentiality and uncertainty about potential etiologies of disease and treatment plans.

The following descriptions differentiate the types of shift reports: (a) Bedside handover or walking rounds: off-going nurse introduces the on-coming nurse to the patient and discusses the plan of care. The patient may listen to the report and ask questions. Individualized goals and patient progress are presented. This helps the on-coming nurse to meet the patient, identify needs, and prioritize for the shift. (b) Taped handover: off-going nurse records the report for on-coming shift; off-going nurses may listen alone. (c) Written handover: the off-going nurse writes the report by hand or on a computer for the on-coming nurse. (d) Real-time oral handover: takes place in a designated location whereby the off-going nurse describes patient information while the on-coming nurse documents information and asks questions; nurses are not at the patients' bedsides for a time interval. Delays in assembling the team may hinder patient care activities. This report may be presented to the entire team as a global nursing report or one to one.

In the United Kingdom, there are two forms of handover. Main handover takes place some distance from patients; team handover follows main handover. Team handover occurs when two to three nurses gather in teams for report (Payne et al., 2000). An example of different forms of shift reports was used by an emergency unit in the United States (Zimmerman, 2006). "Semi-walking" rounds were begun before the starting time of staff nurses. The on-coming charge nurse received report for the off-going charge nurse during walking rounds and made assignments for the next shift. Next, the on-coming direct care nurse received a report from the off-going direct care nurse (Zimmerman, 2006).

Nurses use different strategies to collect and integrate data for shift report. Sources of data are comprised of paper charts, transcribing information from the charts; computerized records, if available; and personalized report sheets using scraps of paper are thought to be more dynamic and consistent with patient events (Hardey et al., 2000). The latter records can be replaced by personal digital assistants or iPad (Strople & Ottari, 2006).

The psychological and social dynamics of a change-of-shift report reveal their importance to nurses' education on direct care strategies, nursing values, and the intricacies and functions of the role of the nurse. Performing a shift report constitutes a test of nursing expertise. If a new nurse is not performing adequately, this is evident during reports (Wolf, 1986a, 1988a). However, bullying, a type of relational aggression, is also evident on observation of change-of-shift reports. Using put-downs or humiliation about a nurse's skills and ability is detrimental to individuals and group culture. Conflicts must be addressed so that a positive work environment flourishes. Zero tolerance is recommended along with education on dealing and coping with bullying (Dellasega, 2009).

Time spent immediately before a report is shaped by the current unit climate. When this time coincides with patient crises, it is very difficult for nurses to accomplish handovers. Nurses may quietly center themselves before beginning the exchange. Others just begin (Armstrong, 1991) the report. Charge nurses, qualified and competent RNs, consistently deliver change-of-shift reports (Flynn, Prufeta, & Minghillo-Lipari, 2010). Whether rotating or permanent, the expertise of nurses in charge of groups of patients and directors of staff contribute much to teamwork and a positive work environment. Variability in the selection of charge nurses and their preparation for the role suggests that standardized orientation workshops need to be implemented during which competencies are developed and effective communication is emphasized. Their compliance with a standardized report format to promote consistency from shift to shift might contribute to patient safety and quality of care. Furthermore, ongoing support of charge nurses by patient care directors after orientation programs provides ongoing mentorship and support for this essential nursing position (Flynn et al., 2010).

INITIATION TO CHANGE-OF-SHIFT REPORT

A change-of-shift report is most often learned on nursing units (Scovell, 2010), not during nursing education programs. Students, new staff members, and part-time contract nurses are socialized to the roles of the nurse and unit characteristics (Scovell, 2010) through the repeated practice of an intershift report. Nursing students frequently witness oral change-of-shift reports in acute care settings and clinical faculty typically insist that students arrive at units in health care institutions early to maximize this opportunity to experience this important part of nursing practice.

However, the quality of teaching and learning varies according to the unit and staff nurses providing a shift report. Skaalvik, Normann, and Henriksen (2010) investigated students' learning during a shift report. Supervising nurses ($n = 11$) and student nurses ($n = 12$) were interviewed; field observations were conducted, and field notes recorded. Students' learning was limited; they wished for a more professional discussion during the report because professional dialogue fostered their learning. Their experiences varied; some were asked to share opinions about care options for specific patients. They noted the practical nature of an oral report; suggestions about patient care were described. Both retrospective and prospective care planning was discussed. The quality of the report fluctuated. Units where oral reports were patient-centered provided opportunities for students to talk about their experiences and receive support of clinical learning. The investigators concluded that the ideal situation involved an oral report that was person-centered and students learned nursing care, shared what they knew, responded to questions about their knowledge, and were socialized into the professional nursing role. The investigators were concerned that opportunities may be missing and limited students' learning of practice routines. Encouraging students to ask questions during real-time handoffs in clinical agencies may prepare and promote their clinical reasoning abilities and begin to develop competencies for change-of-shift reporting (Lim, 2011) and represent an initiation strategy.

Learning the process and content of change-of-shift reports calls for a formal educational program (Manning, 2006) for new RNs and nursing students. Case studies simulate actual clinical situations for new nurses and students. Preparing a simulation experience in which students role-play different roles common to those performed by staff involved in a change-of-shift report may assist students in building confidence with this challenging nursing responsibility. Students' personality traits vary, so creating such an interactive session that matches all students challenges faculty (Lundberg, 2008). The use of SBAR (Situation Background Assessment Recommendation/Request) approach can be used as an initial approach to standardize communication (Ascano-Martin, 2008; Manning, 2006). Some nursing students are learning this format when providing clinical information in health care settings. Furthermore, having students present their patients using change-of-shift structure, content, and process might increase students' self-confidence in giving a report (Ascano-Martin, 2008).

New staff nurses are initiated into the role of the nurse through a change-of-shift report. Their skills and knowledge are revealed during their performance. Each neophyte is tested, corrected, shaped, sanctioned, rejected, or accepted by colleagues (Wolf, 1988a, 1989c). Nurses are either gentle or sarcastic in their comments. Questions are answered and teaching is provided spontaneously and freely (Wolf, 1986a).

ARTISTIC PERFORMANCE OF A CHANGE-OF-SHIFT REPORT

Charge nurses deliver change-of-shift information skillfully. They are masters of the professional jargon of nursing (Wolf, 1989c) and health care, using abbreviations and acronyms and other idiosyncratic health care terms. Their proficiency is evident to nursing students and new nurses in awe of the insider speech used during report.

Experienced nurses' clinical ability is reflected during a change-of-shift report. Their mastery of patient care is shared with new nurses. As skilled clinicians, they teach neophytes about direct patient care skills, technologic equipment, medications, and management of hospital policies and procedures. Their speed of delivery is a feature of skilled performance (Payne et al., 2000).

Nurses' personal style is apparent during a shift report. Their emphasis, tone, and order of delivering information (Staggers & Jennings, 2009) is tailored by their unique preferences, most likely a combination of personality, knowledge, and experience. The report is sacrosanct for nurses as it is a test of clinical expertise. It no longer excludes patients, family members, and other health care providers. However, when bedside reporting started, nurses had to learn to explain some of the insider terminology.

RESEARCH ON CHANGE-OF-SHIFT REPORTS

Research on a change-of-shift report is abundant and has evolved over the last several decades. Many of the investigations selected are qualitative with a more recent pattern of quantitative studies emerging (see Table 5.1). The investigations reveal the different functions of change-of-shift reports, its importance in the culture of nursing practice, strategies for effective shift reports, and some of the interpersonal problems among the nurses. The studies also show an ongoing need to standardize the format and documents used in change-of-shift report and the variability of information presented. Surprisingly, one finding pointed out the lack of information about nursing care during handovers.

CHANGE-OF-SHIFT REPORTS AND SYMBOLS

At a symbolic level, change-of-shift reports persist as an initiation strategy or rite of passage (Wolf, 1986a, 1988a) where new nurses' performance is tested and knowledge, skills, and values are taught by more experienced, skilled colleagues. Despite the labeling of a shift report as a *sacred cow* (Caruso, 2007), shift reports are closely intertwined with professional nursing's culture and dramatizes societal values internalized by the nursing profession (Holland, 1993). They have "special" meaning and ennoble everyday and routine nursing practice (Sherman & Mitty, 2008). Shift report is an important stage for "relationship-centered principles of professional performance...such as how healthcare professionals communicate, make decisions, and collaborate" (Thornby, 2006, p. 267).

TABLE 5.1

Results: Reviewed Citations

Study/Article	Theoretical Basis for Study	Design; Question/ Purpose, Sampling Frame/Size	Independent Variables (IV); Dependent Variables (DV)	Measurement of Variables (Name of Instrument, etc.)	Statistics Used to Answer Research Question	Findings
Walker (1967)	Ritualistic practice as dysfunctional	Descriptive, field study; to study nurses' behavior within an organizational context; the effects of the internal characteristics of the organization upon the hypothesized tendency for ritualistic behavior by nurses	Ritualistic practice of nurses in hospitals: change-of-shift report, temperature, pulse, respiration, and nurses' note procedures; incident reports, interruption and reassignment of nursing activities	Semistructured interviews; taped interviews		Verbal report functioned to transfer latest patient information; to share unique patient information, to talk in order to share responsibilities Redundancy of information Promoted social cohesion of group and opportunity to settle intershift conflicts
Wolf (1986a)	Frame of reference: anthropological, sociological, and nursing literature	Qualitative, ethnography; What actions, words, and objects make up nursing rituals? What are the types of nursing rituals demonstrated by professional nurses caring for adult patients? What explicit or manifest meanings do these rituals have to nurses, patients, and their families, and to other hospital personnel?	Context: Medical nursing unit of large urban hospital to study 1. postmortem care, 2. admission of patients to the hospital and discharge of patients from the hospital, 3. medication administration, 4. bath, handling of excreta and secretions, caring	Participant observation (fieldwork) and field notes, semistructured interviews, event analysis, document analysis		Therapeutic nursing ritual: the bath, bathing patients; postmortem care (context: "do not resuscitate" dilemma); medication administration Occupational nursing ritual: change-of-shift report Patient ritual: admission to the hospital Change-of-shift report occurred repeatedly at specific times and imposed order on easily disordered events of patient units; time suspended (for patient care); functioned as a forum for socialization of nurses into the role of the nurse

for patients with
infectious disease,
and
5. change-of-shift
report

What implicit or
latent meanings are
identified by the
nurses, patients,
and other hospital
personnel, and by the
investigator?
How do nursing rituals
emerge in the context
of postmortem
care, medication
administration,
admission and
discharge procedures,
change-of-shift report,
and the aseptic
practices of nurses,
including the bed bath
and the care of infected
patients?
Informants: nurses,
patients, family
members, hospital
personnel

Worries, complaints, possible errors, and
standards of nursing care described;
shift report represents continuous
coverage and taking on responsibility
for patients

(continued)

TABLE 5.1

Results: Reviewed Citations (continued)

Study/Article	Theoretical Basis for Study	Design; Question/Purpose, Sampling Frame/Size	Independent Variables (IV); Dependent Variables (DV)	Measurement of Variables (Name of Instrument, etc.)	Statistics Used to Answer Research Question	Findings
Richard (1988)	Sensory information and overload and effect on perception of nurses in hospital environment	To determine the percentage of congruence, incongruence, omissions, and omissions resulting in incongruence between intershift reports and actual conditions of patients; convenience sample intershift reports ($N = 57$; 2,952 entries	Congruence, incongruence, omissions, and omissions resulting in incongruence of intershift reports	Data collection sheet (11 predetermined objective items)	Congruence = 70%; omission rate = 11.76%; overall incongruence = 12.36%; two omissions resulting in incongruence is skin condition; significant relationship between mode of report (taped vs. face-to-face) and lack of congruence ($X^2 = 9.24$, $df = 2$, $p = .01$)	Most common omission, intake and output; most common incongruence, IV sites; taped reports more likely than face-to-face to produce omissions, but less likely to produce incongruence
Ekman and Segesten (1995)	Value of oral communication during shift report; ritual as special form of communication (Turner, 1969);	Qualitative, ethnography; 10 oral shift reports	Task allocation of oral shift reports on nursing unit	Fieldwork, participant observation, tape-recorded and transcribed shift reports; field notes		Before report delivery (preliminal phase): reporting nurse—accountable and burdened; receiving nurse—prepared and exhilarated During report delivery (liminal period): reporting nurse—handing over deputed power; receiving nurse—receiving deputed power

	rites of passage (van Gennep, 1960)				After report delivery (postliminal phase): reporting nurse—discharged, relieved; receiving nurse—reincorporated, accountable, but not ready to account Main symbol: deputed power of medical control; process of transferring authority and responsibility; nurses paid minimal attention to nursing care; nursing virtually invisible Reports mainly retrospective
Strange (1996)	Ritual in nursing, ineffective versus valuable; cultural immersion and understanding of symbols in context (Helman, 1990)	Qualitative, ethnography; to identify features and functions of nursing handovers, everyday pattern of nursing practice; nursing staff	Handover functions and symbolic meaning	Participant observation	Rule: report should not be too long; begins with lowest numbered bed and progresses to highest numbered bed; other professionals excluded; report followed by on-coming shift allocating patients to nurses Handover can be considered a ritual with many functions: psychological (protective effect by reducing uncertainty and anxiety); social (group bonding and cohesiveness); identification and management of deviant cases (inappropriate nurse behavior); protective (knowledge that something is being done for patients reported on; helps with feeling of control) Report reveals expressive aspects and key values of nursing culture: obedience to authority and awareness of nurses' position in nursing hierarchy

(continued)

TABLE 5.1
Results: Reviewed Citations (continued)

Study/Article	Theoretical Basis for Study	Design; Question/ Purpose, Sampling Frame/Size	Independent Variables (IV); Dependent Variables (DV)	Measurement of Variables (Name of Instrument, etc.)	Statistics Used to Answer Research Question	Findings
Banks (1999)	Theory of Goal Attainment (King, 1996)	Nonexperimental, descriptive; to describe the structure and content of the intershift report as reported by RNs employed on acute care medicine unit; RNs (N = 59) from medicine units	Structure used to organize intershift report; content conveyed in intershift report	Researcher developed survey including intershift report structure and content, interviews		Some used documents, valued report; report did not always start on time; environment not always conducive to report; frequent interruptions; length of report time 15 to 30 minutes Content: highest communicated: admission diagnosis, reason for admissions, significant findings, procedures, treatments, PRN medication, physical assessments, laboratory data/scheduled tests, respiratory care, change in condition Content items added: reason for admission, problems with giving medication, changes in condition related to nursing interventions, PRN medication outcome, past medical history, results of tests/procedures; much of content medically focused
Manias and Street (2000)	Handover as process of communication	Qualitative, critical ethnography (textual analysis); to examine the practices used by nurses in communicating with other nurses during the handover; part of	Practices nurses use in communicating with other nurses during handover	Professional journaling, participant observation, individual and focus group interview; textual analysis		Handover provided an overview of patients between nurse coordinators and on-coming previous shifts; showed a lack of specific patient information at the bedside Nurses scrutinized nurses and their care and were fearful about their clinical practices; tyranny of tidiness (nurses

larger study in critical care setting; RNs (N = 6)

How do nurses exercise power in their activities and in conversation in the nursing handover? Who is under examination during the nursing handover? When and how are nurses examined during the nursing handover? What practices are more apparent than others while nurses communicate during the nursing handover?

demonstrated ability to maintain patient tidiness); tyranny of business (compulsion to perform physical tasks around patient's bedside or immediate clinical environment); sense of finality (need to complete nursing task before providing verbal account to relieving nurse)

(continued)

131

TABLE 5.1
Results: Reviewed Citations (continued)

Study/Article	Theoretical Basis for Study	Design; Question/ Purpose, Sampling Frame/Size	Independent Variables (IV); Dependent Variables (DV)	Measurement of Variables (Name of Instrument, etc.)	Statistics Used to Answer Research Question	Findings
Hardey et al. (2000)	Use of information in clinical care conceptualizing nursing as a process	Qualitative, ethnography grounded theory; how scraps influence delivery of nursing care: Content and context of patient-focused knowledge constructed through interactions between nursing staff; interviews (N = 34, staff and senior nurses, students, auxiliaries)	Personalized recordings on paper	Nonparticipant observation, tape-recorded handovers, semistructured), document analysis		Main source of nursing scraps: pieces of paper or small handbooks; construction and content of scraps: range from to do lists to complex systems recording diversity of information, body-related tasks, evaluative, emotional, or intuitive statements; proud of skills in constructing scraps; role and use of scraps: main source of information at handover and norm to which new nurses expected to adhere; confidentiality and disposal: personalized nature of scraps, uniquely tailored to meet information needs of individual nurses; not in accordance with priorities for handovers and nursing other records, potential breach of rules of confidentiality
Dowding (2001)	Information content of shift report; theories of information processing (Newell & Simon, 1972); theories of	Experimental, factorial design; to explore the possible way information is processed during the change-of-shift report in acute medical and surgical wards in order to provide evidence	Structure of shift report (retrospective and task-orientated or prospective and patient-focused) (IV); type of information (schema consistent or schema inconsistent)	Amount of information, checklist, total score; plan of care created by expert panel	Two-way analysis of variance	Type of information (retrospective vs. prospective) had significant effect on nurses' ability to plan care; type of information (schema: consistent vs. inconsistent) had significant effect on information accurately recorded; type of shift and schema had significant effect on information accurately recalled

	knowledge organization: schema theory	with which to explore the relevance of the change-of-shift report to nursing practice; RNs (N = 48), 12 subjects in each group	(IV) scenarios constructed for each experimental condition (8); nurses' ability to access appropriate knowledge and plan of care or amount of information accurately recorded about patient during shift report (DV); amount of information subjects accurately recalled after shift report (DV); quality of plan of care constructed (DV)			
Kerr (2002)	Conceptual orientation: Definition: continuity of care. Function: classification and types. Location: office and bedside.	Qualitative and quantitative, inductive: cross-sectional, comparative, case study design, two wards; to gain a better understanding of how handovers operate and to examine the nature of this nurses-to-nurse communication; to analyze handover	Practices and activities of handover; classify and characterize functions of handover; identify some effectiveness and problem criteria	Observation of key events and activities; field notes; interview guide on handover issues (practices, functions, problems, and effectiveness); individual and group interviews	Descriptive statistics on handover functions by case (ward)	Off-going and on-coming staff; three phases: prehandover (preparation for intershift meeting), intershift meeting (report), posthandover (uptake of nursing care by new shift) Handover functions: informational (patient reports, patient updates, family problems), social (supportive, socializing), organizational (planning the shift and patient-to-nurse allocation), educational (teaching, socialization)

(continued)

TABLE 5.1
Results: Reviewed Citations (continued)

Study/Article	Theoretical Basis for Study	Design; Question/ Purpose, Sampling Frame/Size	Independent Variables (IV); Dependent Variables (DV)	Measurement of Variables (Name of Instrument, etc.)	Statistics Used to Answer Research Question	Findings
	Methods: spoken, written, taped	function, particularly more hidden and informal aspects; cases (wards): 1. oncology and hematology specialty with clinic and community ties; 2. three types of surgery: ear, nose, throat; plastic; dental—12 individual interviewees				System of inherent tensions: formal versus informal practices; comprehensiveness versus overload; confidentiality versus family-centered care; single versus multiple functionality
Sexton et al. (2004)	Handover patterns; implicit and explicit functions of handover, inherent problems in process, and various handover styles	Qualitative; to examine content of verbal nursing handover in relation to existing documentation structures in medical ward; handovers on all shifts (N = 23)	Content of verbal nursing handover related to existing documentation structure	Qualitative data analysis: coding structures	Counts, percents	Most reports did not use paper sources of patient information; bed lists with patient name and diagnosis used for notes; 69.5% of information discussed could be incorporated into existing documentation; one-half of remaining information irrelevant to ongoing patient or ward management; reports haphazard and lack clear and concise guidelines

| Pothier, Monteiro, Mooktiar, and Shaw (2005) | Handover methods and process | Quasi-experimental, pilot; to assess the resilience of handover methods; to determine which method is most effective and reliable method of transferring patient information; RNs (N = 5) | Simulated one-to-one handover scenario; 12 fictional patients with relative potential for mortality or morbidity: expert clinician designation of category; each scenario with 21 data points to be handed over; categories: medical history, social history, general nursing data; typed data sheets for each patient (random assignment of fictional patient scenarios, three groups: verbal with no note-taking, written with verbal report with note-taking, sheet, typed sheet with all patient details and verbal report) (IV); accuracy of handover (DV) | Videotaped handovers assessed for data content accuracy by three independent investigators: number of correct data points; number of data points omitted; number of incorrect data points inserted | Loss of data: Verbal with note-taking versus written with verbal and note taking ($p < .001$); verbal with note-taking versus sheet ($p < .001$) | Verbal with no note-taking group: more data loss than written with verbal and note-taking and sheet and verbal groups; highest accuracy sheet with verbal report group Handover sheets with verbal report recommended to increase data transfer during shift report |

(continued)

135

TABLE 5.1
Results: Reviewed Citations (continued)

Study/Article	Theoretical Basis for Study	Design; Question/ Purpose, Sampling Frame/Size	Independent Variables (IV); Dependent Variables (DV)	Measurement of Variables (Name of Instrument, etc.)	Statistics Used to Answer Research Question	Findings
Hays and Wienert (2006)	Patterns affecting role performance through dramaturgic approach: charge nurses and RN staff nurses; performances (shift reports); social action within an expected specific role (Goffman, 1959)	Qualitative, case study: secondary analysis of acted videotaped hospital shift reports to reflect the emotional displays of RNs and to identify commonalities that impact the interactions; 12 shift reports with four charge nurses and 13 staff RNs	Role performance (actors, audience, performance roles, protagonists, antagonist, auxiliary players)	Target Behavior Instrument: 10 observable behaviors to define communication interactions (effective leader behaviors, effective follower behaviors, ineffective follower behavior)	162 behaviors identified	Charge nurse did not exhibit any verbal or nonverbal supporting behaviors of praise, concern, or assurance in behaviors (absence of verbal support to peers or nurse manager) Charge nurse behaviors varied by high-to-low energy levels; single report was different; single individual was different Emphasized necessity of stating goals, the most important task confronting group members, at beginning of change-of-shift report
Yonge (2008)	Shift report is common nursing practice; types of shift report compared; shift report as ritual	Qualitative, ethnography; to describe daily activities of staff, patients, and families in residential adolescent psychiatric word; bring to light what was assumed or taken for granted	Mental health nursing shift report	Participant and nonparticipant observation, interviews, audiotaped shift report, questionnaires, document analysis; domain		Perfunctory written reports left by night shift; day to evening report, most extensive with greatest number of staff present; staff were in favor of verbal, private shift report; pace of report leisure: staying on topic and issue Language used in report facilitated group morale All adolescents had a staff advocate

Author/Year	Purpose/Sample	Focus	Data/Methods	Findings
	about shift report; explore language, perceptions, thoughts, and beliefs of informants regarding shift report; maintained a holistic approach; observe the balance between process and product; patients (n = 13); families of two former patients; nursing staff (n = 14); ancillary staff (n = 17)		analysis; taxonomic analysis; componential analysis (Spradley, 1979)	Report was brief narrative relating previous 8 hours in the life of each patient under staff supervision; statement of global assessment; recitation of staff's judgment of most salient details in support of this judgment; staff spoke in turn Tacit code of conduct; venting necessary prelude to stepping back and regarding a case objectively Stratification of report: main narrative supplied by orator; one or more discursive or digressive subtexts contributed by listeners
Staggers and Jennings (2009)	Qualitative; to describe current content and context of change-of-shift report on medical and surgical unit; to explore whether nurses use computerized support during the change-of-shift report; medical and surgical units (N = 7; N = 13 reports: 53 patients, 38 nurses)	Content and context of change-of-shift reports	Audiotaped reports, field notes	Themes: dance of report or discernible movements between report partners, accompanied by interruptions, distractions, forgetting something, losing one's train of thought; just the facts or exchange of noncontroversial, factual patient data, completed work or treatment work; professional nursing practice or nursing actions, knowledge, reasoned judgments, and instincts combined with care decisions, assessment, observations, decisions; lightening the load (thoughtfulness toward staff, teamwork, bonds, smoothing shift transition)

(continued)

TABLE 5.1
Results: Reviewed Citations (continued)

Study/Article	Theoretical Basis for Study	Design; Question/Purpose, Sampling Frame/Size	Independent Variables (IV); Dependent Variables (DV)	Measurement of Variables (Name of Instrument, etc.)	Statistics Used to Answer Research Question	Findings
						Context: question about how nurse receives the big picture; mostly noisy settings; difficulty locating on-coming nurse to receive report; time consuming; personalized tools or records created (Kardex or interdisciplinary care plan may be used); none used electronic health record; nurses delivered report using their own style, rapid shifts topic to topic, clipped speech, abbreviations and acronyms; interruptions common
Riesenberg, Leitzsch, and Cunningham (2010)	Systematic review process	Systematic review; 95 articles abstracted; 20 in final review	Nursing handoffs	Application of quality of scoring system (Downs & Black, 1998); type of citations reviewed: anecdotal, intervention without control group, abstract, review, cross-sectional, editorial, commentary, qualitative, cohort, and letter		Barrier categories: communication; problems associated with standardization; equipment issues; environmental issues; lack of or misuse of time; difficulties related to complexity of cases or high caseloads, lack of training or education; human factors Strategies for effective handoffs: communication skill development; standardization strategies; technologic solutions; environmental strategies; training and education; staff involvement; leadership

138

| Jukkala et al. (2012) | Quality improvement; threats of poor communication to patient safety | Pilot study; preexperimental; MICU nurses (*n* = 43, baseline; *n* = 34 posttest) | Quality improvement on clinical microsystem, best practices, MICU communication tool; (IV), shift communication (DV) | MICU Shift communication scale, 3 domains: communication openness, quality of information, shift report; 1 = strongly agree, 4 = strongly disagree | Paired *t*-tests; $M = 18.85$ (baseline); $M = 17.71$ (posttest); $t = 2.23, p = .03$ | Significant improvement in communication specific to shift report; differences in subscale total scores statistically significant |
| Maxson, Derby, Wrobleski, and Foss (2012) | Continuity of care, patient safety, nursing handoff, bedside shift change | Descriptive, survey; to determine if bedside nurse-to-nurse handoff increases patient satisfaction with plan of care and increases patient perception of teamwork; to determine if bedside nurse-to-nurse handoff increases staff satisfaction with communication and accountability; staff nurses (*n* = 15); patients (*n* = 60, 30 before and 30 after) | Practice change, implementation of bedside nurse-to-nurse handoff (IV); satisfaction items (DV) | Surveys, patient (five items) and nursing staff (five items) | Wilcoxon rank-sum test: item on patients' being informed of plan of care, $p = .02$; all items significantly different, $p < .05$, with exception of shift report helps nurses prioritize workload, $p = .04$ | Bedside nurse-to-nurse shift handoff had positive impact on patients and nursing staff satisfaction |

Nurses see the change-of-shift report as a critical event for exchanging patient information (Anderson & Mangino, 2006). Expert charge nurses accomplish skilled communication and have vital conversations with on-coming nurses. They signal their gradual taking on of responsibility for the care of patients during and after the report. A comment such as, "I'm not on shift yet; I haven't got the report" (Ekman & Segesten, 1995, p. 1008) illustrates the importance of the completion of the ritual.

Important functions take place during intershift reports as nurses validate nursing decisions, define their role, mentor novice nurses, demonstrate clinical expertise, cope with job-related stress, and shape team cohesiveness. Such social, psychological, and educational functions weave throughout the performance of a shift report (Strople & Ottari, 2006). Nurses who cared for dying patients appreciated shift reports for gathering information and creating expectations that assisted them in planning nursing intervention actions. They shared thoughts and feelings; this supported them emotionally in the care of their dying patients (Hopkinson, 2002). Shift reports implicitly illustrate the emotional labor of nursing.

For years, the language of shift report kept noninitiated, neophyte nurses, nursing students, and patients and families confused about communication interchanges. Even so, the professional jargon of change-of-shift reports endures. However, it has been modified as nurses explain health care terminology, treatment plans, and various circumstances to patients and families during bedside reports.

As the locations where a shift report is performed have changed, so too have the documents associated with it. Nurses' responsibility for patient safety and quality will continue to be evident as electronic health records are more intensively integrated into a shift report. This evolving change explicitly signals nurses' determination to communicate significant information shift to shift on behalf of patient care and to share their cultural beliefs, norms, and values.

SUMMARY

What is surprising about selected literature on change-of-shift reports is the theme demonstrating that little content addresses clinical nursing practices. Investigators have noted that nursing-specific information has been described as being virtually invisible (Ekman & Segesten, 1995) in report content. This invisibility is confirmed by the transitory nature of documents used in shift reports such as scraps (Hardey et al., 2000), nursing care plans, and reports sheets (Athwal et al., 2009). Of similar concern is that nurses' ideas are underestimated (Mason, 2004).

Shift reports are nursing's domain. Many believe that nursing work would be much more difficult without them. Furthermore, nurses have the power to shape their performance, including content and context. Nurses must value shift reports' unique contributions to patient care and work to identify the many contexts that shape that care (McCloughen et al., 2008). To do this calls for carrying out the skilled communication standard of the American Association of Critical Care Nurses so that crucial conversations happen during each shift report (Thornby, 2006). It also calls for collaboration with patients, families, and other health care providers. Bedside reporting and standardized shift report documents seem to foster collaboration.

Clinical performance deficits surfacing during shift reports need to be identified by off-going nurses from the previous shift so that on-coming peers can check and remediate problem areas (Dellasega, 2009; Sims, 2003). Furthermore, nurses need to reflect on their language and tone during reports, challenge assumptions, and eliminate gossip. Demonstrating professional civility and codes of conduct and holding themselves and others accountable (Rushton, 2010) will reset the norms of shift reports. Team collaboration builds trust, and trust most likely positively influences communication. Adopting a need-to-know policy and developing policies and standards for respect, privacy, and confidentiality will result in improving unit morale (Rushton, 2010).

Involvement of staff in changes to shift reports have been described in many studies and related literature. Approval of practice councils and unit staff involve nurses and other nursing staff in shift report changes. Nurses as individuals and groups need to develop self-esteem personally and as a group too and promulgate their power after development of self-esteem at the staff level (Hays, 2003). Changes to shift reports are challenging and need to be evaluated and modified after piloting. Demonstrating nurses' capability and accountability for evidence-based changes of shift reports and the connection of reports with outcomes will confirm their importance.

Standardization of care processes is essential to improving staff, patient, and family satisfaction (Sims, 2003). Standardization can also result in decreased overtime and costs. However, examples of standardization of content vary (Bosek & Fugate, 1994), so that evidence-based content needs to be investigated, piloted, and revised.

Improving the work environment using rapid cycle process improvement could be used for a change in an intershift report. For example, the beginning of shift changes includes an overview, whereby the off-going charge nurse communicates to the entire on-coming shift significant issues on the unit, writes reminders on the staff white board, compliments, and provides comments (Sims, 2003). Next, direct caregivers meet in smaller groups to discuss their patients' situations. Subsequently, team huddles take place every 3 to 4 hours to exchange updates on patient status and concerns between nurses and other nursing staff (Anderson & Mangino, 2006). Huddles can include patient safety briefings whereby information is shared to keep staff informed, anticipate needs, and plan accordingly (Manning, 2006). Standardization of shifts can build teamwork, as seen in a unit when all staff moved to 12-hour shifts (Kalisch, Begeny, & Anderson, 2008; Wooten, 2000).

The nonlinear, complex nature of nursing work is lived by nurses. One example revealed nursing care activities reported on at the end of each shift (Potter et al., 2004). Attention to human factors engineering demonstrated the work of one RN caring for six patients through a nurse's cognitive pathway. The complex patient care process was depicted in a task analysis and an intricate list of observed activity with interruptions analyzed. This example of nursing work from the perspective of disruptions in the nursing process not only points to the likelihood of errors, but also dramatizes the complexity of communicating relevant information during subsequent shift reports. Combining human factors engineering techniques and qualitative observation methods showed the dynamic nature of nursing care across time and illustrated the importance of nurses' cognitive work. Nurses are challenged during every change-of-shift report to condense their shift experience accurately, thus representing the current status of their patients and revealing important personal, unit, institution, and social imperatives.

6

Nursing Ceremonies: Transitions Into and in Celebration of Professional Nursing Work

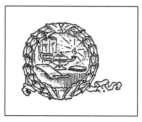

Nurses conduct ceremonies of transition into the profession and in celebration of many academic and professional achievements. As evidence of social and cultural processes with distinctive structures, ceremonial events mark important points in nurses' professional lives and represent life transitions through ritual performance. Schools of nursing do not conduct white coat ceremonies, common to medical and dental schools (Goldberg, 2008; Huber, 2003; Peltier, 2004). In contrast, the nursing culture has created distinctive nursing ceremonies. Although the features of the performance have evolved, nursing ceremonies persist and formalize nursing students' movement from non-nurse through important milestones of nursing education programs. Pinning ceremonies also mark the end of nursing education programs and the achievements of graduating students. New knowledge has been imparted and learned and new power is absorbed as students move from marginal to full status following licensure.

Many other observances of nurses' accomplishments are carried out in addition to different rites of passage (Van Gennep, 1960). For example, nursing service departments in hospitals celebrate National Nurses Week, which occurs each year in May, in commemoration of Florence Nightingale's birthday and in praise of nurses' contributions to health care. Publications such as the journal, *Nursing Management*, have recognized visionary leaders at their Congress (Holmes Regional Medical Center and Palm Bay Community Hospital, 2006). Other events observe nurses' achievement of distinguished status, such as inductions to Sigma Theta Tau International, the American Academy of Nursing, and the Academy of Nursing Education. Within professional organizations, there are award ceremonies at annual meetings. Eastern Nursing Research Society honors research expertise for neophyte and seasoned investigators through its awards committee and by honoring colleagues at annual meetings. The American Nurses Association and the Academy of Medical-Surgical Nurses also celebrate distinguished nurses and schools, and programs of nursing applaud notable alumni. Such ceremonies convey nurses' respect for the accomplishments of colleagues.

Passages distinguishing changes in the life cycle of individuals as well as changes in social role not only are marked by overt expressions of recognition during ceremony, but also have ritual importance. They separate individuals from formal roles and observe their achievement and transition to new ones. Rites of passage acknowledge nursing students' persistence through trials inherent in nursing programs; they have made it through various steps.

They defer initially to the wisdom of other nurses (after Grimes, 2000) and ultimately gain status. The norms, values, and beliefs of professional nursing culture have not only been transmitted, but internalized.

Awards or gifts given during ceremonies highlight the celebratory aspects of these ritual performances, whether they are pins or other objects symbolizing new roles or achievements. These objects represent achievements of professional nursing. For nursing program graduates, wearing them reveals that previous dependencies and reliance on nursing faculty, staff nurses, and preceptors are relinquished. New mentors will appear.

The classic theory of Van Gennep (1960) on rites of passage depicts the transition of individuals across and within cultures as they transition from one role to another. Those individuals metaphorically stand on a threshold or limen, and progress through the phases of separation, transition, and incorporation (Van Gennep, 1960). Nursing rituals of transition or rites of passage communicate and renew the basic values of the culture. Socialization into the role of the nurse is begun for new nurses or advanced in complexity for experienced nurses.

NURSING CEREMONIES AS INITIATIONS

Nursing faculty have many opportunities to transmit the culture of professional nursing to students. They often do not label or list their attempts to do so, but in fact accomplish a powerful acculturation in classrooms, clinical settings, laboratories, and offices. "A school is still a privileged institution for the transmission of culture. In the scholastic environment, the teacher is the principal actor who transmits culture. In a sense, the professor is the faithful guardian of culture, the heir" (Padilha & Nelson, 2011, p. 190). Ideally and gradually, students internalize the beliefs, values, and norms of the culture of nursing; this is marked by ceremonies celebrating rites of passage.

Faculty and administrators of nursing programs have prolonged contact with students and this opportunity serves their implicit agenda of sharing and transmitting the nursing culture, the chief value of which is respect for human dignity. They are also the first filter for the profession. Nursing's important work with people demands that schools attract and retain persons of highest character (Jowett, 1997).

It is the initial responsibility of nurse academics to help students learn the traditions and history of professional nursing. The sense of professional identity begins with students understanding the cultural context of the profession; their appreciation can be facilitated through the programmatic messages in nursing ceremonies. Not to hold these formalities nor teach nursing history could allow the profession to risk its own sense of connectedness and cohesiveness, dramatized by the loss of new graduates to long-term careers (Madsen, McAllister, Godden, Greenhill, & Reed, 2009). Rites of passage ceremonies highlight "a moment of personal and social change as worthy of collective attention" (Grimes, 2000, p. 133).

Capping Ceremonies

Capping ceremonies in the United States recognized nursing students' movement from probationary status to more secure places in their nursing education program and anticipated profession. Capping ceremonies were solemn occasions. "Big sister" and "little sister" relationships were often set up to ease students' transition through mentoring activities. Students in diploma, associate degree, and baccalaureate programs were awarded caps, and customarily each year caps changed in some way to symbolize that students were closer to the goal of professional nurse (Hawkins & Redding, 2004). Often, stripes were added to caps on completion of each year of study. Student caps were replaced by different style caps after graduation, worn only by graduates of that nursing program. Students also wore distinctive uniforms consistent with school or program. This practice continues presently.

Caps gradually disappeared in schools of nursing and clinical agencies; nursing caps' elimination was attributed to concerns with medical asepsis and their inconvenience when worn in clinical settings. Despite being pinned to female nurses' hair by "brain patches" (Kleenex and bobby pins), they got caught in curtains around patients' beds and would fly off during codes. Some were very difficult to launder, such as the incredibly beautiful "double frill" worn by graduates of the Philadelphia General Hospital School of Nursing. This cap is similar to one worn by a Florence Nightingale disciple, Alice Fisher, seen in an oil painting portrait circa 1888 and located at the Bates Center for the Study of Nursing History at the University of Pennsylvania School of Nursing. Caps are still worn in other countries, but rarely by nursing staff in clinical agencies in the United States. Older nurses are still proud of their caps and know exactly where they are stored ("What happened to the cap," n.d.).

Changes in nurses' dress have paralleled the elimination of caps, perhaps beginning with nurses wearing pantsuits. Clinical attire is now very practical with casual looking scrubs or more functional uniforms used in schools of nursing and clinical settings. Not only have white uniforms virtually disappeared, but "clinic" shoes have been replaced by sneakers and clogs. Nursing service departments have begun to standardize the color of scrubs worn by RNs. RNs on staff at the Hospital of the University of Pennsylvania wear navy blue scrubs (Jost & Rich, 2010), designating them as *the* nurse. The importance of the title *registered nurse* is lived in this institution. Similarly, nursing students' more informal attire, when compared to students of the 1950s, is consistent with that of many professional nurses. Wearing these uniforms also reflects their transformation to neophytes of the profession of nursing.

Professional Nursing Ceremonies

Professional nursing or commissioning ceremonies have been inaugurated recently to help students mark the evolution from student to professional nursing student; they are not exclusive to programs in the United States (Padmanabhan,

2003). These events replace or are alternatives of capping ceremonies. A "commitment-to-nursing ceremony" was inaugurated at the College of St. Mary in Omaha, Nebraska (Hawkins & Redding, 2004). For several years a similar ceremony has been held at La Salle University in Philadelphia, Pennsylvania. The aim of both is to illustrate nursing's professional values and education and the seriousness of the nurse's role in society and to congratulate students on reaching this milestone or crossing a threshold.

The program presented at the professional nursing ceremony at La Salle University, a Brothers of the Christian Schools university, initially was a response to incivility among nursing students. Faculty were concerned and recognized that they needed to help students internalize the values of the profession. A teaching plan (or guideline) now serves as the foundation for the images and the script presented during the ceremony. The worldwide reach of the Brothers of the Christian Schools is briefly explored. Images of nurses at war and at work in different settings are included along with a brief history of nursing programs at La Salle University.

Candles and flowers are placed on a table and correspond to the university's colors; a baccalaureate hood, with the apricot color designating nursing degrees, is draped on the table. Images of symbols of the La Salle Christian Brothers, Florence Nightingale, registered nurses, and selected nursing symbols from organizations across the world are incorporated into the visual presentation.

Brief examples of nursing history as antecedents to current nursing practice are narrated and may help students expand their "thinking, professional courage and identity...and bring cohesiveness to everyday occurrences" (LeMaire quoting Herrmann, 2002). Following the recitation of a revised version (Fowler, 1984; Grainger, 2011; Newland, 2011; Nursing Programs, La Salle University [Appendix A]; Ocean County College, 2008) of the original Nightingale Pledge (Gretter, 1893 [Appendix B]), students' foreheads and hands are anointed with aromatic oil and a prayer is offered for each as a blessing: *Blessed are the minds that advance the wonders of science and the hands that heal the wounded, sick, and vulnerable.* A faculty member and the former dean revised the Nightingale Pledge to fit with current practices and nurse autonomy, patient confidentiality, and a commitment to patients first (Erickson & Millar, 2005; McBurney & Filoromo, 1994). Students also receive a small pin in the shape of a nursing lamp, symbolizing nursing knowledge.

Rising Senior Ceremony

Another example of a celebration in honor of nursing students reaching senior year placement began with students realizing that their nursing program had few ceremonies of professional socialization (Lee, Idczak, Moon, & Brown-Schott, 2006). Students selected Virginia Henderson's description of an effective nurse as a theme for the ceremony: strong minds, healing hands, and compassionate hearts. With faculty support, they planned and carried out the ceremony, presented a certificate to each senior, and narrated readings on the important work of nursing. With each year the ceremony became more elaborate, recognizing students and building bonds among them (Lee et al., 2006). Storytelling and lessons from history presented by students could be incorporated into this event in celebration of nursing's contributions to society (McAllister, John, & Gray, 2009).

This ceremony parallels earlier recognition of students' progression in programs when stripes were added to their nursing caps. For instance, a striping ceremony program is available in a nursing archive (University of Oklahoma, School of Nursing, 1951). Additionally, one response to a query on striping ceremonies posted on Allnurses.com clarified the practice:

> The striping ceremony is dedicated to 1st year nursing students as recognition of completing a very demanding year. The stripe I believe was originally meant to be placed on the cap. Each school would have their own unique stripe. The tradition has been continued in some schools even though the caps have not. It is a meaningful recognition to the students and an opportunity to share this accomplishment with family/friends. I would like to know if anyone out there has a school that still practices this beautiful ceremony. (Allnurses.com, n.d.)

Another respondent noted that a striping ceremony was held in the Philippines as recently as June 2011.

Pinning Ceremonies

Pinning ceremonies scheduled before university commencement exercises mark students' completion of undergraduate nursing programs (Hallett, 2010, pp. 180–181). Since the elimination of the nursing cap as a unique symbol of a nursing program, each nursing pin stands as its chief representation and a symbolic object of the transition to the role of RN. The nursing faculty assembles at the event in support of students and in recognition of this passage.

Typically, nursing pinning ceremonies recognize the achievement of a significant miestone in a professional nurse's life. Completing an approved program is linked in the United States with formal certification of the graduate with the respective state board of nurse examiners. That certification and successful passing of the NCLEX-RN® transitions each graduate to RN status.

Nursing pinning ceremonies typically follow a format (U.S. Federal News Service, Including U.S. State News, 2012). Speeches and the actual pinning performance dramatically convey the status of ritual to the event. Graduates cherish their pins and faculty members advise them to wear the symbol of the program with pride.

Pins are cast in unique designs for each nursing program (Reed, 2009). They are made of a variety of metals and are more or less ornamented. Both decorative and sacred images on nursing pins stand for a specific school and its representation of educated nurses. They symbolize and legitimize the completion of a program of studies, keeping outsiders out and insiders in (Chapman, 1983).

The roots of nursing pins could be in the fourteenth century when trades with common interests formed guilds signified by symbols. Universities and schools followed with the implicit meaning of the symbol referring to the "exclusivity, prestige, protection, fidelity, training and standards" of nurse education programs (Connecticut Nursing History Vignettes, n.d.; Rode, 1989). In contrast, a precursor to the nursing pin may have occurred when Queen Victoria presented a brooch to Florence Nightingale in 1855 in recognition of her work in the Crimean War (Nursing Connection citing Kentucky Nurses Association, 2006). However, it is more likely that pins or badges were developed to indicate graduates who completed a course of study or a nurse training program:

> Before long, however, the public's growing recognition of the worthiness of nurses, but its ignorance of what constituted legitimate nurse's training for that time period, inadvertently allowed some unscrupulous individuals to imitate the trained nurses' demeanor and attire. Disturbed by the imposters' infringement and exploitation, some graduating classes of trained nurses took matters into their own hands; they designed and adopted "class pins" to wear on their uniform. While the adoption of class pins was an attempt to thwart deception by others and to differentiate competent from incompetent practitioners, the wide variations in the pins from class to class in a single school ultimately negated the intended purpose. To overcome that limitation, the administrators of schools of nursing began awarding their graduates an official and distinctive pin that uniquely represented their institution. Commonly the pins were also engraved on the reverse side with the graduate's name and date of graduation. In some cases the pins were gifts from the school's Board of Managers; other times the graduates purchased them from the school. (Connecticut Nursing History Vignettes, n.d.)

The first nursing pin in North America signifying a training school was that of the Bellevue Hospital Training School in New York City. Tiffany and Company designed the pin in 1880 to preserve the identity and uphold the standing of Bellevue Hospital Training School and demonstrate the wearer's character as well as achievement (New York Health and Hospitals Corporation, n.d.). In addition, the development of the nursing pin may have been an antecedent to nurse registration legislation (Connecticut Nursing History Vignettes, n.d.).

Even now, wearing a school's or program's pin is a privilege. Nursing pins are sentimental treasures for nurses. Most wear their pins on lab coats not on scrubs.

Nurse Practitioner Ceremony

The transition of experienced, acute care, baccalaureate-prepared nurses to primary care nurse practitioner roles challenges many nurses. In recognition of the need to honor and bless this role transformation, faculty members developed the Willow Ceremony (Burman, Hart, Conley, Caldwell, & Johnson, 2007). The ceremony's intent was to welcome nurse practitioner students into the world of advanced nursing practice. The choice of the willow tree symbolized the strength, grounding, and flexibility of advanced practice nurses.

According to faculty, the program presents the history and ethical basis of the nurse practitioner movement. Welcomes and words of wisdom were offered along with a willow branch and a poem on initiation into advanced practice roles. Students have appreciated the ceremony and faculty have continued to focus on ethical values as the program content evolved.

No matter which ritual event takes place and in whatever form, these ceremonies mark the transition of students from nonprofessional to professional or advanced practice nurse. The enactment allows the culture of nursing to be illuminated.

NURSING CEREMONIES IN CELEBRATION OF NURSES' WORK

Celebratory ceremonies have been part of modern nursing's traditions. They have recognized exemplary role models in nursing and shared accomplishments with the nursing community at local, regional, national, and international levels. The transformative power of ceremonial performances conveys the values of professional nursing culture to individuals and groups (McAllister et al., 2009). Ceremonies help nurses solidify their professional identity following completion of educational programs. Some confer full citizen status in a cultural group and provide rights, duties, privileges, powers, and liabilities to members (Murdock et al., 1961).

Various types of nursing ceremonies can be classified as bonding, blessing, status declaration, community celebration, and incorporation or integration events. Perhaps, the actions that are performed can be described as rites or ritualized gestures. Many have been constructed solely by organizations, perhaps recognizing nurses' need to "revise existing rites and compelling new ones" as they "sense the need for bodily and collective ways of making meaning" (Grimes, 2000, p. 3). These celebratory rituals belong in and to the nursing culture, contextualized by history, academic institutions, the characteristics of health care organizations, and the nature and mission of professional nursing organizations. Some interpret the tribal nature of professions and units in health care agencies and their rituals negatively, at the same time they value signaling the importance of and propagation of ceremonial activity within institutions (Brooks & Brown, 2002).

Organizational rituals are comprised of symbolic practices and communal rites, symbolizing shared meaning, as they are enacted during ceremonies (Smith & Stewart, 2010). They transmit values and beliefs of an organization and confirm status. They also function in organizations to demonstrate and reinforce social order and commitment and manage anxiety (Smith & Stewart, 2010).

Academy Induction Ceremonies

The establishment of organizations named as nursing academies demonstrates the commitment of many nurses to honoring colleagues who stand out. For example, the American Academy of Nursing (AAN), dedicated to serving the public and the nursing profession by advancing health policy and practice through generation, synthesis, and dissemination of nursing knowledge, is recognized as a prestigious group of nurses (AAN, n.d.). The AAN selects fellows each year who have made outstanding contributions to nursing and health care and will have an impact on the Academy. Selection is based on sponsor nominations, applicant statements, and the AAN Fellow Selection Committee. Fellows are also recognized as Living Legends, honoring their extraordinary and continuing contributions to the nursing profession throughout careers (AAN, n.d.). Honorary fellows are also named by virtue of extraordinary contributions to nursing and health care, otherwise ineligible for membership as a regular fellow. Each year AAN celebrates the induction of new members at the annual meeting during the Living Legends and Induction Ceremony.

The American Academy of Nurse Practitioners (n.d.) recognizes select nurse practitioners as fellows and applauds their accomplishments and contributions to the advancement of the nurse practitioner role. The National League for Nursing (NLN) also established the NLN Academy of Nursing Education. Its purpose is fostering "excellence in nursing education by recognizing and capitalizing on the wisdom of outstanding individuals in and outside the profession who have contributed to nursing education in sustained and significant ways. Fellows...provide visionary leadership in nursing education and in the Academy support the vision of the National League for Nursing" (NLN, n.d.). The annual meetings and induction ceremonies of the American Academy of Nursing, the American Academy of Nurse Practitioners, and the Academy of Nursing Education perform rites of integration. The ceremonials are inclusive and public (Beyer & Trice, 1987) and demonstrate the significance of professional nursing organizations.

Health Care Organization Ceremonies

For decades, nursing service organizations have recognized nursing staff annually, events typically coinciding in the United States with National

Nurses Week and Florence Nightingale's birthday. Many times, these events have been aimed at fostering team building. They also function as a way for nurses to empower themselves. They demonstrate the cohesion and mutual goals of the nursing staff.

In institutions with 24-hour coverage, nurse administrators have instituted creative ways to reach all staff during that week with a series of events and with refreshments. The amount of ritual performance varies, but many times guest speakers present on relevant topics and certificates of achievement are distributed to stand-out nurses. A shortened version of the press release about the Veterans Administration Maryland Health Care System's (2012) observation of National Nurses Week With Awards Ceremony is found in Appendix C.

This time has also been set aside to celebrate nurses who achieved certification or recertification, typically earned by examination and a reported number of clinical hours completed in a specified clinical area. Examples include certifications as emergency nurse, oncology nurse, or critical care nurse. Another example of recognition during an annual Nightingale Award Ceremony was the commendation of mentors for sponsoring new graduates and designating the mentor of the year. At another time, these mentors were honored through a half-day program set aside for them, including speaker presentations (Pinkerton, 2003).

A Certified Nurses Day was recently established to recognize RNs across the globe who contribute to better patient outcomes. On March 19 each year, nurses who are certified in their specialty are honored (ANCC, 2012b). Certified Nurses Day honors nurses worldwide who contribute to better patient outcomes through national board certification in their specialty.

Achieving certification recognition indicates advancement in the profession. An RN license allows nurses to practice. Certification builds on knowledge gained at licensure and confirms nurses' advanced knowledge, skill, and practice. Employers, certification boards, education programs, and health care providers celebrate and publicly acknowledge nurses earning and maintaining the highest credentials in their specialty.

OTHER RECOGNITION EVENTS

Speas (2004) advocated for peer recognition of fellow nurses; her suggestions included tangible recognition with certificates and simple objects such as pins and thank you cards. Correspondingly, a three-hospital system developed the SHINE (Scottsdale Healthcare's Investment in Nursing Excellence) voluntary program. The aim of the program was to promote professional development and evidence-based practice among nurses and to recognize and reward their accomplishments (Post & Righi, 2010). Points were awarded for engaging in professional education, community, team-centered activities, and organizational commitment (years of service). Patient safety improvements, professional development achievements, and recruitment and retention strategies resulted, generated by nursing staff. The SHINE awards ceremony recognized SHINE recipients and made monetary awards and contributions to continued professional development such as journal subscriptions or conferences.

The Magnet Recognition Program of the American Nurses Credentialing Center (ANCC) has succeeding in generating considerable interest on the part of nursing service organizations desiring to establish their institutions as recipients of the Magnet award (Smith, 2003). It is evident that this mark of excellence is worth the time, effort, and costs associated with submitting an application and hosting site visitors, expended by aspiring nursing service departments. Magnet institutions evidence a commitment to ongoing excellence for nursing departments in the context of the larger health care institution. The "forces of magnetism" shape organizational culture as nursing service departments aimed at retaining Magnet recognition once awarded.

Magnet recognized institutions are known as excellent places for nurses to work. Nurses' work is supported in order to achieve the highest quality of care and is autonomous, collaborative, accountable, and self-regulating (Stolzenberger, 2003). Magnet institutions have increased RN retention and satisfaction, decreased vacancy and turnover rates, and lowered nurse burnout (ANCC, 2012a, 2012c). The Magnet experience strengthens the infrastructure of nursing organizations, is a mark of pride for acute and long-term care agencies, and builds respect and understanding among the nursing staff (Stolzenberger, 2003). Many organizations create annual events to celebrate Magnet status and use the opportunity to recognize outstanding nurses.

Celebratory rituals can function as rites of renewal (Beyer & Trice, 1987) in the nursing service organization. They may accomplish hidden, expressive consequences for the department. For example, publicity about outstanding nurses spreads good news about the department and provides public recognition of individual accomplishments, thus motivating others to do the same (Beyer & Trice, 1987). Nursing departments can also take credit for individual accomplishments.

In a study on ritualistic ceremonials in the National Health Service of the United Kingdom, Brooks and Brown (2002) studied ceremonies as perpetuating barriers among work groups and considered if ceremonies could be changed, what positive outcomes would occur to effect organizational change. The predominantly phenomenologic investigation used semistructured interviews, observation, and document analysis as data sources. Ceremonies functioned to accomplish cultural change in organizations. They suggested that ceremonies might help organizations incorporate or consolidate new ways. They found that ceremonies of preservation preserved the demarcation between groups or subcultures, such as the standard times that drugs are administered and the "them and us" attitudes between night- and day-shift nurses. They classified types of ceremonies of preservation: belonging, continuity, resistance/questioning, conflict reduction, integration, resistance, degradation, belonging, and continuity. Examples of ceremonies of change included reclassifying ancillary and portering staff as care assistants and talking-up the crisis of the competitive threat of a nearby large hospital. Types of ceremonies of change posed were: passage, degradation renewal, sense-making, challenge, integration, and legitimization. Brooks and Brown (2002) suggested that organizational ceremonies, if modified, could foster the implementation of change and the success of that change.

When new employees join health care organizations, they learn about the nursing department's celebrations. By participating in the rituals as they take place during the first year of employment, they are incorporated into the culture of the organization. For them, the celebrations serve as rites of passage.

SUMMARY

Nursing excellence is honored by many nursing service organizations across the United States. The greatest attribute of these awards and ceremonies is that nurses are recognizing expert colleagues who exemplify the best performance of the profession. In contrast, some argue for removal of dysfunctional ceremonies. They suggested that such action could result in positive organizational change by proposing that an opportunity exists for managers to change ceremonies carefully and influence cultural change (Brooks & Brown, 2002). Nonetheless, nursing ceremonies in praise of excellence are sustained as valuable professional events.

Many descriptors of excellence are available in the narrative summaries describing nurses' contributions to the profession presented during ceremonies. Attributes of excellence have been established (Jasovsky et al., 2010) and will continue to be added to and refined. Most impressive is that the important values of the profession are sustained and that the bar of achievement continues to be moved to higher levels, all with excellent patient care as the ultimate outcome. The rituals of celebration performed by professional nursing organizations and health care institutions' nursing service departments can be classified as bonding, status-declaring, and incorporating rituals (after Grimes, 2000, p. 43). In this way, nursing notifies its public about the expert clinicians, educators, researchers, administrators, and leaders.

In contrast to organizational rituals and ceremonies, a ritual was created to honor nurses who died as a celebration of their service. The Kansas State Nurses Association offers The Nightingale Tribute, including a downloadable brochure, for nurses to use to commemorate the life of a nurse. The poem "She Was There" by Duane Jaeger, RN, MSN is published in this brochure with the intent of reading the poem during a memorial service.

The pronoun is changed to make it gender appropriate. Family members are consulted about the reading of a poem and the placing of white roses with the deceased nurse and a symbol of appreciation for a colleague.

It is also critical that the ceremonies preceding completion of nursing education programs continue. Students benefit from learning the history of nursing, values, and culture of professional nursing. Rites of transition and incorporation, or rites of passage, acknowledge the distinct attributes of the culture of nursing. They function to involve students in its norms and hopefully help and motivate them to remain in practice after graduation and licensure. Consequently, nursing will continue to provide new practitioners to sustain its greatest contribution to society, nursing care of patients, families, and communities.

APPENDIX A

Nightingale Pledge Revised

I solemnly promise before God and all present
to live my life honorably and morally and to practice my nursing profession faithfully. I will never intentionally harm anyone in my care and work determinedly to practice nursing safely. I will never take or knowingly administer any harmful drug or therapy. I will do all in my power to maintain and elevate the standard of my profession by active engagement, a commitment to caring, continuing education, and mentorship of new nurses and nursing students.
I will keep all health and personal information of patients and families confidential as I practice my calling.
I will work collaboratively and respectfully with all health care providers and devote myself to the welfare of those committed to my care.

Source: Nursing Programs, La Salle University.

APPENDIX B

Nightingale Pledge

I solemnly pledge myself before God and in the presence of this assembly:
To pass my life in purity and to practice my profession faithfully.

I will abstain from whatever is deleterious and mischievous, and will not take or Knowingly administer any harmful drug.

I will do all in my power to maintain and elevate the standard of my profession and will hold in confidence all personal matters committed to my Keeping and all family affairs coming to my Knowledge in the practice of my profession.

With loyalty will I endeavor to aid the physician, in his work, and devote myself to the welfare of those committed to my care.

Written under the leadership of Lystra E. Gretter, principal of the Farrand Training School for Nurses at Harper Hospital, Detroit, Michigan, in 1893.

APPENDIX C

VA Maryland Health Care System Observes National Nurses Week With Awards Ceremony

May 5, 2012

The Veterans Affairs (VA) Maryland Health Care System will observe National Nurses Week (May 6-12) with an awards ceremony on May 7, at 3 p.m. in the auditorium at the Baltimore VA Medical Center. Janet D. Allan, PhD, RN, FAAN, dean of the University of Maryland School of Nursing, will deliver the keynote address on the future of nursing. During the ceremony, nurses will be honored with the VA Secretary's Award for Excellence in Nursing and the 2012 DAISY Award.

"We consider our nurses—the largest of our workforce at more than 900 strong, of which 700 are RNs and Nurse Practitioners—to be the compassionate backbone of our health care system," said Dennis H. Smith, director of the VA Maryland Health Care System. "We are thrilled to honor the dedicated men and women who have mastered the art and science of caring for our nation's heroes with compassion. No other health care professional is closer to the Veterans we serve than VA nurses. Our patients rely on them for their compassion, and the VA relies on them for setting the highest clinical care standards."

The VA Secretary's Award for Excellence in Nursing consists of three major categories: Excellence in Nursing, Advancement of Nursing Programs by a Medical Center or Health Care System Director, and Advancement of Nursing Programs by a Medical Center or Health Care System Nurse Executive.

EPILOGUE

Nursing Rituals

Nursing rituals are discoverable in narratives describing elements and situations of nursing culture. They appear in anecdotes and stories of professional nursing practice, many of which are not recorded. Nursing rituals accentuate the importance of the events they represent. They do not necessarily function nor are always carried out to deal with the communal anxiety or the crises of professional nursing. Nurses do not label or link nursing rituals with crises. However, some of nursing's direct care rituals might be viewed as a response to crises, in that nursing practice often involves caring for patients who need to be cured and healed and who suffer and die.

Nursing rituals do, however, go to the root of each nurse's being and there a nurse who contemplates ritual action might discover something profoundly communal and shared (Turner, 1969). Nursing rituals dramatize events of significance to nurses. Their performance is marked by formality and a certain amount of repetitive or even rigid activities. Their symbols signify shared values and meanings, such as respect for human dignity, the intention to serve persons requiring nursing services, nursing's close, elemental, and almost primal association with care of the human body in intimate and personal space, the need to respond to those in need who call for a nursing response, the imperative to do good and avoid harm, the imposition of order on disorder, and the value of being compassionate. Moreover, many of nursing's direct care rituals are symbolically represented by the metaphor of "hands-on" (Engebretson, 2002).

Rituals are often called sacred or described as consecrated behavior. Consider the rituals of bathing patients or performing postmortem care. In each of the hands-on, direct care nursing rituals, the biogenic or life-giving mode described by Halldorsdottir (1991) can be said to operate. Nurses as ritual performers are open to patients, receptive to them, compassionate, and share energy with them as they bathe patients, such as in intensive care units, or care for patients as they are dying, or even after death during postmortem care. As the last care nurses give patients, nurses try to protect family members from witnessing the traces of suffering evident on their loved ones' bodies. They honor patient preferences above those of the family, clean the patient, and make them ready for the next transition, depending on advanced directives, last will and testaments, and family requests.

Although the interpersonal caring ritual does not always involve nurses' physical presence, it can still be considered a hands-on, direct care nursing ritual. The nursing occasion, moment, meeting, or situation involves nurses' caring consciousness and takes place in a zone or territory whereby nurses place their needs secondary to patients'. The interpersonal caring ritual is the most essential performance of nursing practice, in that all nursing care follows this initial stage and all that follows is described as nursing care.

Nurses' presence and engagement with patients establish interconnections as nurse–patient relationships unfold. Nurses are receptive, intentional, respectful, and caring. Often, the shared consciousness between nurses and patients brings out the whole of the interconnected human experience: mind, body, and spirit.

Nurses as witnesses and ritual participants share in important transitions in patients' lives, such as being hospitalized, admitted to a nursing home, or needing home care or hospice. They may be the only witness to patients' experiences, particularly when all family members have died or are not present. Also, as nurses pass on their personal responsibility for patient care to the next nurse during a change-of-shift report, they consistently carry out intensely important communications through the fundamental nurse–patient relationship and with other members of the health care team. Nursing rituals similarly mark important events in the lives of nursing students and RNs, in the instances of professional rites of passage, and celebratory events when awards are given for excellent practice, research, and teaching. Celebratory rituals help nurses rejoice as a community about their work and one another's contributions to patients, families, and health care.

There are some nursing activities that have been and continue to be labeled as rituals, but they have either never been rituals or at least have lost their status as such; an example is taking temperatures at routine times during a 24-hour cycle. Or, they have changed dramatically and have lost their correspondence with commonly held nursing values. They are considered ritualistic, redundant, mindless, and unscientific, and because of these judgments call for elimination or at the very least, disregard. Nurses who write about the uselessness of nursing rituals are very critical; their arguments are sometimes convincing. Some of these so-called rituals have never been "true" rituals; most likely their activities have been ritualistic. Others have been transformed as

TABLE E.1

Types of Ritual	Ritual Examples	Ritual Elements	Values
Therapeutic, comforting, healing patient	Interpersonal caring ritual	Authentic presence, gaze, intention, consciousness, words of greeting, touch, body position of nurse (intimate and/or private space), embodied nurse, embodied patient	Beneficence, respect for human dignity, privacy, freedom from risk of injury, autonomy over one's body (self-determination), justice (treat all patients fairly), disclosure, clinical autonomy
Therapeutic, purification, comforting, healing patient	Bathing ritual	Authentic presence, intention, hands-on, words, equipment, embodied nurse, embodied patient	Beneficence, respect for human dignity, privacy, freedom from risk of injury, autonomy over one's body (self-determination), justice (treat all patients fairly), disclosure
Therapeutic, comforting, healing patient, family, and friends	Postmortem care ritual	Authentic presence, intention, consciousness, hands-on, words, equipment (intimate and/or private space), embodied nurse, embodied patient	Beneficence, respect for human dignity, privacy, freedom from risk of injury, autonomy over one's body (self-determination), justice (treat all patients fairly), disclosure
Therapeutic, healing patient, protection from harm	Medication administration ritual	Authentic presence, intention, consciousness, hands-on, words, equipment (intimate and/or private space), embodied nurse, embodied patient	Beneficence, respect for human dignity, privacy, freedom from risk of injury, autonomy over one's body (self-determination), justice (treat all patients fairly), disclosure
Socialization; passing on and taking over continuous responsibility and accountability: covering, watching out, carrying out duty; witnessing	Change-of-shift report ritual	Special language, intention, consciousness, words, role modeling, teaching	Beneficence, do not harm, respect for human dignity, societal trust, surrogate for patient, family, friends, justice (treat all patients fairly), clinical autonomy
Rite of passage	Nursing students' rituals of transition	Transmission of values, consciousness, words, role modeling, teaching	Beneficence, respect for human dignity, privacy, autonomy over one's body (self-determination), justice (treat all patients fairly)
Rite of passage	Professional nursing ritual for students: transition	Transmission of values, consciousness, words, role modeling, teaching	Beneficence, respect for human dignity, justice (treat all students fairly)
Recognition of expertise and achievement	Group celebration	Transmission of values, consciousness, words, role modeling, teaching	Beneficence, respect for human dignity, justice (treat all nurses fairly), clinical autonomy

the profession has changed, but persist nonetheless even as objects, gestures, and words have evolved and through the gradual incorporation of technology, scientific findings, changes in nursing staff assignment through differentiated tasks, and so forth.

The mere mention to nurses that nursing rituals appear in everyday practice situations and are present in ordinary nursing care activities does not come as a surprise to direct care nurses or those who are managers and directors. They accept the existence of ritual without using a theoretical framework or operational definition of it. They acknowledge them as real. Some might realize that a ritual just occurred, stop, and say, "I guess that was a ritual." Nursing practice situations in which rituals are performed transform the character of nursing work and define it with special meaning. Their performance is not common but extraordinary. In this way, just some of the exceptional nature of nurses' work is illustrated by ritual symbols.

Nursing rituals do not negate scientific results or evidence; they coexist and coevolve with science. However, they may not always function in harmony with scientific findings. This is because much of ritual is latent and inferred and requires a certain amount of faith or belief, almost automatically making nursing rituals questionable in some scientific circles. In addition, nurse scientists may not have paid a great deal of attention to exploring and describing nursing rituals. These considerations, along with a dearth of empirical evidence, rituals' relative invisibility, and the inference needed to substantiate ritual outcomes, reinforce rituals as suspect. One counter to this argument that partially supports their existence is the maxim that in every human activity there is belief, art, science, and ritual. Another is that when one ritual disappears, another takes its place, suggesting that humans must have rituals in their lives.

Table E.1 classifies the rituals examined in this book according to type, provides specific examples, delineates ritual elements, and proposes ethical values that orient these selected nursing rituals.

Nursing rituals are passed on by demonstration, reminiscence, and storytelling. They are conscious and intentional. Nursing rituals ennoble nursing practice in spite of what nurse watchers, as outsiders, may see as mundane and routine. Direct care nursing rituals originate in caritas or compassion. They and rituals of socialization, rites of passage, and celebration provide order and clarity in times of change and crisis. They tie nurses together as a cultural group and with patients and family members.

Nursing rituals are rooted in values of significance to humanity. Similar to other cultural groups, nursing rituals arise from the need for nurses to symbolize, make meaning, create community, and deal with the many mysteries of nursing work. They also link metaphysical with physical and past nursing life and practice with the present, and as such will persist.

GLOSSARY

Abject: Defiled; degraded.

Acculturation: Cultural modification of an individual, group, or people by adapting to or borrowing traits from another culture (Merriam-Webster, n.d.).

Adverse event: Injury resulting from medical intervention related to a drug (Bates et al., 1995, p. 29).

Antiritualism: Individuals who revolt against rituals, against established hierarchical systems of religion (Douglas, 1982, p. 4).

Apnea: Absence of breathing.

Art: Quality, production, expression, or realm according to aesthetic principles of what is beautiful, appealing, or of more than ordinary significance.

Asystole: Absence of heartbeat.

Barcode/eMAR: System providing integrated scanning of barcoded medications with the patient's electronic MAR; access to eMAR and laboratory test results; opportunity to check correctness of medications after scanning, verify correct patient after scanning patients' identification band; and text page or mail members of the interdisciplinary team (Eisenhauer et al., 2007).

Bath: A centerpiece of body care for nursing (Lawler, 1991); an assessment opportunity; typically procedural, objective, if not objectifying and clinical (Lawler, 1991, p. 41).

Bedside report: Walking rounds during which off-going nurses report to on-coming nurses about patients in the presence of the patient for the discussion of plans of care; provides a synchronized exchange of information aimed at patient safety, quality of care, accountability, and teamwork (Murray, 2009); allows for questioning (Costello, 2010). Off-going nurse introduces on-coming nurse to patient: explicit transfer of responsibility; opportunity to reassess patients' goals (Manning, 2006). Patient, staff, and physician satisfaction increases, according to many reports.

Belief: Way of explaining the world, including people's behavior (Strange, 2001, citing Abercrombie et al., 1988).

Belief system: The fundamental assumptions, ideas, and expectations that underlie a culture and that generate the range of practices and norms within it.

Beneficence: The doing of active goodness, kindness, or charity, including all actions intended to benefit others. Not all acts of beneficence are obligatory, but a principle of beneficence asserts an obligation to help others further their interests. Obligations to confer benefits, to prevent and remove harms, and to weigh and balance the possible goods against the costs and possible harms of an action are central to bioethics. Beneficence may include four components: (a) one ought not to inflict evil or harm (sometimes called the principle of nonmaleficence); (b) one ought to prevent evil or harm; (c) one ought to remove evil or harm; and (d) one ought to do or promote good (Miller-Keane, 2003).

Bodywork: Direct care involving washing, eating, grooming, dressing, and sleeping; closely associated with traditional caring roles assigned to women in our culture; represented by practical knowledge (Lawler, 1991).

Caring moment, caring occasion: A caring occasion occurs whenever the nurse and a patient come together with their unique life histories and phenomenal fields in a human-to-human transaction. The coming together in a given moment becomes a focal point in space and time. It becomes transcendent whereby experience and perception take place, but the actual caring occasion has a greater field of its own in a given moment. The process goes beyond itself, yet arises from aspects of itself that become part of the life history of each person, as well as part of some larger, more complex pattern of life (Watson Caring Science Institute, n.d.).

Caritas: Latin for charity.

Ceremony: Organized performance associated with cultural groups that dramatizes rites of passage and other transitions, milestones, and progressions of stages; characterized by an organized, systematic approach to the event through a prescribed succession of rites; accompanied by symbols.

Charge nurse: A qualified, competent leader who oversees patient care on a shift and serves as a resource for fellow staff; role includes overseeing patient care, providing complete and accurate documentation to minimize the potential for legal issues, and managing and promoting positive staff interactions; clinical skills include clinical/technical, critical thinking, organization, and human relations. Important if communicating a change-of-shift report (Flynn et al., 2010).

Clinical event: Unexpected change in patient condition that does not result in a patient transfer and is not associated with a nursing protocol (Clancy, Delaney, Morrison, & Gunn, 2006). For example, the common complications leading to failure-to-rescue events are pneumonia, shock or cardiac arrest, upper gastrointestinal bleeding, sepsis, deep pain thrombosis. Nurse-to-nurse communication of clinical events may be precursors to failure-to-rescue and thus patient complications: drop in hemoglobin and hematocrit, low blood pressure, fever, and pain are precursors of complications (Carrington, 2012, p. 87).

Communitas: A spirit of unity; a human bond; social alienations are suspended during ritual and displayed as communitas (Driver, 1998, p. 162).

Culture: Consists of whatever it is one has to know or believe in order to operate in a manner acceptable to its members (Goodenough, 1964).

Death watch: A vigil beside a dying person; sitting beside a dying patient; looking after a dying person.

Difficult patients: Those whom nurses perceive consume more nursing time than reasonable for their condition, those who act helpless, impede the work of nursing staff with complaints, do not cooperate with therapies, demand special privileges, make insulting remarks, violate rules, fail to cooperate with requests, play one staff member against another, fail to comply with regimens, use threats toward staff to get their needs met (Wolf & Robinson-Smith, 2007); behavior violates social norms of patient unit.

Dirty work: Occupational activities involving disgusting, degrading, or shameful tasks (Shaw, 2004, p. 1033); messy and stigmatizing occupations perform this labor (Shaw, 2004, p. 1033 citing Hughes, 1971); taboo, hidden from public view (Lawler, 1991, p. 4). Nurses use concealment by doing work behind closed doors or screens (Lawler, 1991, p. 46).

Electronic health record: Computerized documentation of patient information in digital format including demographic, health history, radiologic and laboratory data, etc.

Embodied: Represented in bodily or material form.

End-of-life care: Focuses on care during the process of dying and death by providing comfort when a cure is no longer feasible.

Error: In dosage terms, given in excess of total number of times ordered by prescriber (Maricle et al., 2007); failure to give an ordered dose (Barker et al., 2002).

Error, commission: Unintentional health care errors; accidental administration of a dose of medication that was not ordered, etc.

Error, deteriorated medication: Use of expired drugs or improperly stored drugs (Berdot et al., 2012, p. 2).

Error, improper dose: Administration of a dose that is greater than or less than the amount ordered by the prescriber, or administration of duplicate doses to the patient (Bohomol et al., 2009, p. 1263); any dose of preformed dosage units that contained wrong strength or number (Barker et al., 2002).

Error, omission: Unintentional health care errors: accidental failure to administer ordered medication to a patient; failure to give ordered dose if no attempt made to administer dose (does not include patient refusal, withheld due to policy, or contraindication); failure to administer an ordered dose to a patient before the next scheduled dose (Bohomol et al., 2009, p. 1263).

Error, physicochemical incompatibility: Simultaneous administration of two or more medicines via same manifold, for example, triple lumen central venous catheter, with resultant inactivation of drug or formation of toxic compounds (Tissot et al., 1999, p. 354).

Error, unauthorized drug: Administration of a drug product in a different dosage than ordered by the prescriber (Bohomol et al., 2009, p. 1263); administering medication that was not ordered for a patient (Maricle et al., 2007).

Error, wrong administration technique: Inappropriate procedure with improper technique used in administration of medicine; use of different technique from one prescribed, improper use of medical device, injection in wrong part of body, and crushing extended-release tablets (Tissot et al., 1999, p. 354).

Error, wrong dose form: Administration of a drug product in a different dosage form than ordered by the prescriber (Barker et al., 2002; Bohomol et al., 2009, p. 1263).

Error, wrong dose preparation form: Incorrect dilution or reconstitution, mixing drugs physically incompatible and inadequate product packaging (Berdot et al., 2012, p. 2).

Error, wrong route: Administration of medication different from prescribed route (Barker et al., 2002).

Error, wrong time: Administration of medication outside a predefined time interval from its scheduled administration time (Bohomol et al., 2009, p. 1263).

Failure to rescue: Clinicians' inability to save hospitalized patients' lives when they experience a complication (a condition not present on admission) (Clarke & Aiken, 2003, pp. 42–43).

Huddles: Team events for problem solving and updating the plan. Anyone can call for a huddle to deal with new issues, added complexities, unusual circumstances, or any need to adapt the earlier plan. Huddles occur frequently throughout the health care system and many times throughout the day (U.S. Department of Defense, n.d.).

Human Factors Engineering (HFE): Combined techniques from the sciences of industrial engineering, ergonomics, and mathematics used to analyze clinical care processes and restructure patient care delivery; used to perform patient safety analysis (Potter et al., 2004, p. 101).

Initiation: Formal admission to a social group; passing from one social status to another.

Interpersonal: Existing or occurring between two persons.

Intersubjective: The relationship between two people who meet and who may share cognition and consensus.

Intimacy: An act or expression serving as a token of familiarity in an atmosphere of privacy.

Intimate health care: Private, professionally close health care interventions.

Liminal: Refers to a threshold as individuals separate from a previous world, transition, and become incorporated in a new world (van Gennep, 1960).

Liminality: State of being on a threshold; demarcated or separated from the social structure but displaying *communitas* or the human bond and an area of common living (Driver, 1998, after Turner, 1967).

Magic: Practices reflecting confidence in the ability to manipulate supernatural forces (Murdock et al., 1961).

Medication, prophylactic: A prophylaxis is a measure taken to maintain health and prevent the spread of disease. Antibiotic prophylaxis refers to the use of antibiotics to prevent infections.

Meeting: The purposeful encounter of nurse and patient where there is a goal in mind. Nurse and patient meet in a nursing situation (Paterson & Zderad, 1976).

Myths: Traditional or legendary stories, usually concerning some superhuman being of some alleged person or event, with or without a determinable or legendary story that is concerned with deities or demigods and the creation of the world and its inhabitants (*Webster's Encyclopedic Unabridged Dictionary of the English Language*, 1989).

Near miss: Impending error; error would have occurred if nurse did not intervene.

Nonmaleficence: Principle of bioethics that asserts an obligation not to inflict harm intentionally; useful in dealing with difficult issues surrounding the terminally or seriously ill and injured. Some philosophers combine nonmaleficence and beneficence, considering them a single principle (Miller-Keane, 2003).

Norms: Explicit or implicit social expectations and informal rules that derive from and operationalize societal values. Unlike values, norms prescribe and regulate specific forms of behavior (Dictionary of the Social Sciences in Politics & Social Sciences); a group's agreed upon set of unwritten rules (Strange, 2001, citing Abercrombie et al.).

Nursing certification: One of two processes in which a professional organization formally recognizes the competence of a nurse to practice a subspecialty of nursing. A process in which the professional organization or association verifies that a person who is licensed has met the standards for specialty practice specified by the profession. The purpose of certification is to assure other professionals and the public that the person has mastered the skills necessary to practice a particular specialty and has acquired the standard body of knowledge common to that specialty (Free Dictionary, n.d.).

Nursing as form of lived dialogue: Nursing is a particular form of intersubjective relating; nursing is a dialogical mode of being in an intersubjective situation; it is communication in terms of call and response (Paterson & Zderad, 1976, p. 23).

Nursing situation: A shared lived experience in which the caring between nurse and patients enhances personhood (Boykin & Schoenhofer, 2001, p. 13). It is the repository of nursing knowledge and the context for knowing nursing (Boykin & Schoenhofer, 2001, p. 17). The nursing situation develops when one person presents self in the role of offering professional services of nursing and the other presents self in the role of seeking, wanting, or accepting nursing services (Boykin & Schoenhofer, 2001, p. 17).

Palliative care: Interdisciplinary care aimed at improving patients' quality of life through holistic relief of suffering using symptom management (Hodo & Buller, 2012, p. 30).

Palliative sedation: Medications that relieve intractable distress, such as terminal delirium, but do not hasten death (Hodo & Buller, 2012, p. 31).

Personal care: Washing, bathing, skin care, personal presentation, dressing and undressing patients (Royal Commission for Long Term Care, 1999).

Personal hygiene: The physical act of cleaning the body to ensure that the skin, hair, and nails are maintained in optimum condition (Downey & Lloyd, 2008 citing Department of Health, 2003).

Phenomenal: Perceptible by the senses or through immediate experience.

Placebo: Any drug or treatment given to appease the patient, rather than to elicit a specific therapeutic response; placebo effect is any nonspecific therapeutic intervention used to elicit physiologic or psychologic effect...any action or remedy not specifically indicated for a particular disease; placebogenic response is the resulting action that takes place within the patient (Blair, 1996, p. 13).

Pollution: Defilement (Douglas, 1975), uncleanness.

Pollution rules: Impose order on experiences; prohibit contact; applied to products or function of human physiology (blood, excreta, etc.); when violated, are sanctioned by grave or trivial sanctions (Douglas, 1975, pp. 53, 55).

Postmortem care: Last office; after-death care; care of the body performed after death that follows institutional procedures and policies and includes cleansing, dressing wounds, positioning of the body, etc.

Presence: Intersubjective and intrasubjective energy exchange with a person, place, object, thought, feeling, or belief that transforms sensory stimuli, imagination, memory, or intuition into a perceived meaningful experience (Gilje, 1992, p. 61); openness and receptivity to the other; being in one place and not the other; being there and being with another; part of holistic caring approach that involves integration of mind, body, and spirit (Gilje, 1992).

Profane: Diverted from the sacred; debased; defiled; unholy.

Relational aggression: Use of psychologic and social behaviors rather than physical violence to cause harm (Dellasega, 2009, pp. 52–53); bullying is a type of relational aggression.

Rights, Five: Medication error procedure taught for many years: right patient, drug, dose, route, and time.

Rite: Standard rite is a symbolic act that draws its meaning from a cluster of standard symbols (Douglas, 1975, p. 102); formal or ceremonial act or procedure prescribed or customary in religious or other solemn use; particular form or system of religious or other ceremonial practice; liturgy; any customary observance or practice; formal or ceremonial act or procedure prescribed or customary in religious or other solemn use; denotes specific enactments located in concrete times and places; refers to a set of actions intentionally practiced and widely recognized by members of a group; rites are differentiated, even segregated from ordinary behavior (Grimes, 2000, p. 28); relatively elaborate, dramatic, planned set of activities that combine various forms of cultural expressions and that often have both practical and expressive consequences (Beyer & Trice, 1987, p. 6). Acts displayed during ceremony; classified as animistic (belief in the existence of individual spirits that inhabit natural objects and phenomena), dynamistic (based on the concept of power), sympathetic (based on belief in the reciprocal action of like on like, of opposite on opposite, of container and the contained, of the part and the whole, of image and real object or real being, or word and deed), positive (volitions [wishes] translated into action), direct (produces results immediately without intervention by any outside agent), contagious (natural or acquired characteristic are material and transmissible through physical contact of over a distance), negative (taboos or prohibitions not to act), and indirect (vow, prayer, or religious service sets into motion some autonomous or personified power such as a deity who intervenes on behalf of the performer of the rite) (van Gennep, 1960, pp. 4–9). Rites are activities that change; they are handed down and evolve as flowing processes (Grimes, 2000, p. 12).

Rites, enhancement: Ceremonial activities that enhance the personal status and social identities of organizational members (Beyer & Trice, 1987, p. 15).

Rite of passage: Bring about the passage of an individual from one cultural state or social status to another in the course of a life cycle (Turner, 1967); passage from one world to the other whereby an individual separates, transitions, and is incorporated into another world (van Gennep, 1960).

Ritualism: Heightened appreciation of symbolic action manifested in the efficacy of instituted signs, and sensitivity to condensed symbols (Douglas, 1982, p. 8). Behavior which has a special significance to the actor rather than orientation toward achieving organizational goals. Behavior is directed toward tasks contributing to goal achievement; behavior satisfies some psychological need of the individual, for example, compulsive cleanliness, status needs, or reduction of anxiety (Walker, 1967).

Ritualist: One who performs external gestures without inner commitment to the ideas and values expressed (Merton, 1968, p. 131); a student of or authority on ritual practices or religious rites; one who practices or advocates observance of ritual, as in religious services.

Ritualization: A particular cultural strategy of differentiation linked to particular social effects and rooted in a distinctive interplay of a socialized body and the environment it structures (Bell, 1992, p. 8); used to communicate with humans and others; display what words interpret; the making up of behavior routines (Driver, 1998, p. 15).

Ritualize: Make into a ritual (*Webster's Encyclopedic Unabridged Dictionary of the English Language*, 1989); activity of deliberately cultivating or inventing rites (Grimes, 2000, p. 29).

Routine: Observable relationship pattern occurring among individuals on a consistent basis that describes, explains, and predicts the uniqueness of the group as the members interact and respond to their environment (after Denham, 1995).

Sacred: Society's relation to the gods, religious behavior, aspect of prescribed social behavior (Douglas, 1975 citing Smith, p. 49).

Sentinel event: An unexpected occurrence involving death or serious physical or psychologic injury, or the risk thereof. Serious injury specifically includes loss of limb or function. The phrase "or the risk thereof" includes any process variation for which a recurrence would carry a significant chance of a serious adverse outcome. Such events are called "sentinel" because they signal the need for immediate investigation and response. The terms *sentinel event* and *medical error* are not synonymous; not all sentinel events occur because of an error and not all errors result in sentinel events (The Joint Commission, 2011).

Stereotype: The process of simplifying and standardizing a conception or image and investing it with special meaning that is held in common by members of a group (after *Webster's Encyclopedic Unabridged Dictionary of the English Language*, 1989).

Stigma: A mark of shame or discredit.

Symbol: Recalls or represents something by possession of analogous qualities or by association in fact or thought; smallest unit of ritual which still retains the specific structure in a ritual context; examples of symbols are objects, activities, relationships, events, gestures, and spatial units in a ritual situation (Turner, 1969, p. 19); exhibit the properties of condensation, unification of disparate referents, and polarization of meaning; symbols are multivocal; referents drawn from many domains of social experience and ethical evaluation; referents tend to cluster around opposite semantic poles (Turner, 1969, p. 52); generally designates the combination of a sign (a word, graphic, gesture, image, etc.) with its meaning (tree, honesty, patriotism, etc.), although there is considerable variation in usage (Dictionary of the Social Sciences in Politics & Social Sciences).

Taboo (tabu): Nonreligious rules of conduct, especially those concerned with pollution in order to distinguish them from the rules of holiness protecting sanctuaries, priests, and everything pertaining to gods; shunned (Douglas, 1966). The ritual avoidance of a person, place, or thing. The word "taboo" is Polynesian in origin, but it has come to designate prohibitions in many cultures. The concept has figured prominently in the anthropological tradition (Dictionary of the Social Sciences in Politics & Social Sciences).

Traditions: Handing down of statements, beliefs, legends, customs, and so forth, from generation to generation, especially by word of mouth or practice (*Webster's Encyclopedic Unabridged Dictionary of the English Language*, 1989); practices or behaviors passed from one generation to the next; acknowledge the contributions of predecessors with an eye toward the future (Stewart-Amidei, 1994).

Transpersonal: To go beyond one's own ego and the here and now, as it allows one to reach deeper spiritual connections in promoting the patient's comfort and healing (Watson Caring Science Institute, n.d.).

Transpersonal caring: Attends to the human center of both nurse and patient, the one caring and the one being cared for; it embraces a spiritual, even metaphysical dimension of the caring process; it is concerned with preserving human dignity and restoring and preserving humanity in the fragmented, medical cure dominated systems (Watson citing Watson, 1988, p. 177).

Terminal delirium: Displayed as intractable symptoms indicating suffering of the imminently dying person and manifested by confusion, anxiety, agitation, or restlessness (pulling on clothing or sheets) near the end of life; dread, anger, tension, somatic complaints (shortness of breath, nausea, and diarrhea), grimacing, moaning, and agitation (Matzo, 2004, p. 507).

Vigilance, professional: State of scientifically, intellectually, and experientially grounded attention to and identification of clinically significant observations/signals/cues; calculation or risk inherent in nursing practice situations and readiness to act appropriately and efficiently to minimize risks and to respond to them (Meyer & Lavin, 2005, p. 2).

Wrong time error: Administered more than one hour before or after the specified time; administered at different time from prescribed or predefined time (Barker et al., 2002; Tissot et al., 1999).

REFERENCES

Abercrombie, N., Hill, S., & Turner, B. S. (1988). *Dictionary of sociology*. London, UK: Penguin.

Academy of Medical Royal Colleges. (2008). A code of practice for the diagnosis and confirmation of death. Retrieved from http://www.aomrc.org.uk/publications/statements/doc_view/42-a-code-of-practice-for-the-diagnosis-and-confirmation-of-death.html

Academy of Medical-Surgical Nurses. (n.d.). Practice/Research: Position Statements. Medication errors. Retrieved from http://www.medsurgnurse.org/cgi-bin/WebObjects/AMSNMain.woa/1/wa/viewSection?s_id=1073744079&ss_id=536873229&tName=positionsMedicationErrors

Achterberg, J., Dossey, B., & Kolkmeier, L. (1994). *Rituals of healing*. New York, NY: Bantam Books.

Ahluwalia, S. C., Gill, T. M., Baker, D. I., & Fried, T. R. (2010). Perspectives of older persons on bathing and bathing disability: A quantitative study. *Journal of American Geriatrics Society, 58*, 450–456.

Allison, T. G., Miller, T. D., Squires, R. W., & Gau, G. T. (1993). Cardiovascular responses to immersion in a hot tub in comparison with exercise in male subjects with coronary artery disease. *Mayo Clinic Proceedings, 68*, 19–25.

All Nurses. (n.d.). Role of nurses: Bed bathing patient in the hospital. Retrieved from http://allnurses.blogspot.com/2011/06/role-of-nurses-bed-bathing-patient-in.html

Allnurses.com. (n.d.). Striping ceremony: Response to question by SNSCCC, December 15, 2005. Retrieved from http://allnurses.com/first-year-after/striping-ceremony-133852.html

Almerud, S., Alapack, R. J., Fridlund, B., & Ekebergh, M. (2008). Caught in an artificial split: A phenomenological study of being a caregiver in the technologically intense environment. *Intensive and Critical Care Nursing, 24*, 130–136.

Alvesson, M., & Skoldberg, K. (1994). *Interpretation and reflection: Philosophy of science and qualitative method*. Lund, Sweden: Studentlitteratur.

American Academy of Nurse Practitioners. (n.d.). Fellows program. Retrieved from http://www.aanp.org/fellows-program

American Academy of Nursing (AAN). (n.d.). About AAN. Retrieved from http://www.aannet.org/about-the-academy

American Nurses Credentialing Center (ANCC). (2012a). *Benefits*. Retrieved from http://www.nursecredentialing.org/Magnet/ProgramOverview/WhyBecomeMagnet

American Nurses Credentialing Center (ANCC). (2012b). *Certified Nurses Day*. Retrieved from http://www.certifiednursesday.org

American Nurses Credentialing Center (ANCC). (2012c). Forces of magnetism. Retrieved from http://www.nursecredentialing.org/Magnet/ProgramOverview/Historyofthe MagnetProgram/ForcesofMagnetism

Anderson, C. D., & Mangino, R. R. (2006). Nurse shift report: Who says you can't talk in front of the patient? *Nursing Administration Quarterly, 30,* 112–122.

Antai-Otong, D. (2008). *Psychiatric nursing: Biological & behavioral concepts* (2nd ed.). Clifton Park, NY: Thomson Delmar Learning.

Arman, M. (2007). Bearing witness: An existential position in caring. *Contemporary Nurse, 27*(1), 84–93.

Armstrong, N. (1991). How to assess your unit before you take report. *American Journal of Nursing, 91*(2), 57.

Arndt, M. (1994). Nurses' medication errors. *Journal of Advanced Nursing, 19,* 519–526.

Aronson, J. K. (2009). Medication errors: Definitions and classification. *British Journal of Clinical Pharmacology, 67,* 599–604.

Ascano-Martin, F. (2008). Shift report and SBAR: Strategies for clinical postconference. *Nurse Educator, 33,* 190–191.

Athwal, P., Fields, W., & Wagnell, E. (2009). Standardization of change-of-shift report. *Journal of Nursing Care Quality, 24,* 143–147.

Austin, S. (1996). Missed DNR order. *AJN, 96*(2), 55–56.

Babies Hospital of the City of New York. (1889). Points for daily reports. *The Nightingale, 4*(2), 3.

Baldwin, L., & McGinnis, C. (1994). A computer-generated shift report. *Nursing Management, 25*(9), 61–64.

Banks, C. B. (1999). Structure and content of the intershift report. Master's thesis, Christopher Newport University. Ann Arbor, MI: UMI. UMI# 1395625.

Barker, K. N., Flynn, E. A., Pepper, G. A., Bates, D. W., & Mikeal, R. L. (2002). Medication errors observed in 36 health care facilities. *Archives of Internal Medicine, 162,* 1897–1903. Retrieved from www.archintermed.com

Barrick, A. L., Rader, J., Hoeffer, B., Sloane, P. D., & Biddle, S. (2008). *Bathing without a battle: Person-directed care of individuals with dementia* (2nd ed.). New York, NY: Springer.

Bates, D. W., Cullen, D. J., Laird, N., Peterson, L. A., Small, S. D., Servi, D., … Leape, L. L. (1995). Incidence of adverse drug events and potential adverse drug events: Implications for prevention. ADE Prevention Study Group. *Journal of the American Medical Association, 274*(1), 29–34.

Beattie, S. (2006). Post-mortem care. *RN, 69*(1), 24ac1–24ac4.

Beeber, L. S., Canuso, R., & Emory, S. (2004). Instrumental inputs: Moving the interpersonal theory of nursing into practice. *Advances in Nursing Science, 27,* 275–286.

Bell, C. (1992). *Ritual theory, ritual practice*. New York, NY: Oxford University Press.

Benjamin, D. M. (2003). Reducing medication errors and increasing patient safety: Case studies in clinical pharmacology. *Journal of Clinical Pharmacology, 43,* 768–783.

Benner, P. (2000). The wisdom of our practice. *American Journal of Nursing, 10,* 99–195.

Benton, D. (1993). Quality, research and ritual in nursing. *Nursing Standard, 25*(7), 29–30.

Berdot, S., Sabatier, B., Gillaizeau, F., Caruba, T., Prognon, P., & Durieux, P. (2012). Evaluation of drug administration errors in a teaching hospital. *BMC Health Services Research, 12*(60). Retrieved from http://www.biomedcentral.com/1472-6963/12/60

Berlau, D. J., Corrada, M. M., Peltz, C. B., & Kawas, C. H. (2011). Bathing as a potential target for disability reduction in the oldest old. *American Journal of Public Health, 101,* 200–201.

Berman, A., Snyder, S. J., McKinney, D. S. (2011). *Nursing basics for clinical practice*. Boston, MA: Pearson.

Berry, A. (1986). Knowledge at one's fingertips. *Nursing Times,* December 3, 56–57.

Beyer, J. M., & Trice, H. M. (1987). How an organization's rites reveal its culture. *Organizational Dynamics, 15*, 5–24.

Biley, F. (2005). Invisible knowledge. *Nursing Standard, 19*(23), 17–18.

Biley, F. C., & Wright, S. G. (1997). Towards a defense of nursing routine and ritual. *Journal of Clinical Nursing, 6*, 115–119.

Blair, D. T. (1996). The placebogenic phenomenon: Art in psychiatric nursing. *Journal of Psychosocial Nursing & Mental Health Services, 34*(8), 11–15. Retrieved from ProQuest Central.

Blaiss, M. S. (2007). Part II: Inhaler technique and adherence to therapy. *Current Medical Research and Opinion, 23*, S13–S20.

Blank, F. S. J., Tobin, J., Macomber, S., Jaouen, M., Dimoia, M., & Visintainer, P. (2011). A "back to basics" approach to reduce ED medication errors. *Journal of Emergency Nursing, 37*, 141–147.

Blouin, A. S. (2011). Improving hand-off communications: New solutions for nurses. *Journal of Nursing Care Quality, 26*, 27–100.

Bohomol, E., Ramos, L. H., & D'Onnocenzo, M. (2009). Medication errors in an intensive care unit. *Journal of Advanced Nursing, 65*, 1259–1267. doi: 10.1111/j.1365-2648.2009.04979.x

Bosek, M. S., & Fugate, K. (1994). Intershift report: A quality improvement project. *MEDSURG Nursing, 3*, 128–132.

Bosk, C. L. (1980). Occupational rituals in patient management. *New England Journal of Medicine, 303*(2), 71–76.

Bourdieu, P. (1977). Outline of a theory of practice. *Cambridge Studies in Social Anthropology, 16*.

Bourdieu, P. (1990). Was heibt sprechen? Die Okonomie des sprachlichen Tausches. *Braumuller, Wien.*

Bourdieu, P. (1992). *The logic of practice.* Stanford, CA: Stanford University Press.

Bowman, G. (1986). Curbing routine and ritual. *Nursing Times, 82*(31), 43–45.

Boykin, A., & Schoenhofer, S. O. (2001). *Nursing as caring: A model for transforming practice.* Sudbury, MA: Jones & Bartlett.

Brady, A-M., Malone, A-M., & Fleming, S. (2009). A literature review of the individual and systems factors that contribute to medication errors in nursing practice. *Journal of Nursing Management, 17*, 679–697. doi: 10.1111/j.1365-2834.2009.00995.x

Brennan, C. W., Prince-Paul, M., & Wiencek, C. A. (2011). Providing a "good death" for oncology patients during the final hours of life in the intensive care unit. *AACN Advanced Critical Care, 22*, 379–396.

Bright, M. A. (1990). Therapeutic ritual: Helping families grow. *Journal of Psychosocial Nursing and Mental Health Services, 28*(12), 24–29.

Brooks, I., & Brown, R. B. (2002). The role of ritualistic ceremonial in removing barriers between subcultures in the National Health Service. *Journal of Advanced Nursing, 38*, 341–352.

Brown, C. J. (2009). Self-renewal in nursing leadership: The lived experience of caring for self. *Journal of Holistic Nursing, 27*(2), 75–84. doi: 10.1177/0898010108330802

Burman, M. E., Hart, A. M., Conley, V., Caldwell, P., & Johnson, L. (2007). The Willow Ceremony: Professional socialization for nurse practitioner students. *Journal of Nursing Education, 46*(1), 48.

Burr, M. (1906). The care of the dead. *British Journal of Nursing, 37*, 270–271.

Campbell, I. R., & Illingworth, M. H. (1992). Can patients wash during radiotherapy to the breast or chest wall? A randomized controlled trial. *Clinical Oncology, 4*, 78–82.

Carlton, G., & Blegen, M. A. (2006). Medication-related errors: A literature review of incidence and antecedents. *Annual Review of Nursing Research, 24*, 19–38. Retrieved from ProQuest Central.

Carrington, J. M. (2012). The usefulness of nursing languages to communicate a critical event. *CIN: Computers, Informatics, Nursing, 30*(2), 82–88.

Carroll, S. M. (2004). Nonvocal ventilated patients' perceptions of being understood. *Western Journal of Nursing Research, 26*, 85–103.

Caruso, E. M. (2007). The evolution of nurse-to-nurse bedside report on a medical-surgical cardiology unit. *MEDSURG Nursing, 16*, 17–22.

Catanzaro, A. M. (2002). Beyond misapprehension of nursing rituals. *Nursing Forum, 37*(2), 17–27.

Cayleff, S. E. (1987). *Wash and be healed: The water-cure movement and women's health.* Philadelphia, PA: Temple University Press.

Center for Life Enrichment. (2009, October). Preventing medication errors. Retrieved from www.tcle.org/docs/Preventing_Medication_Errors.ppt

Centers for Disease Control and Prevention. (1983). Acquired immunodeficiency syndrome (AIDS): Precautions for health-care workers and allied professionals. *MMWR, 32*, 450–451. Retrieved from http://wonder.cdc.gov/wonder/prevguid/p0000351/p0000351.asp

Centers for Disease Control and Prevention, Department of Health and Human Services. (2003). Physicians' handbook on medical certification of death. Retrieved from http://www.cdc.gov/nchs/data/misc/hb_cod.pdf

Centers for Disease Control and Prevention. (2012). Guidelines for safe work practices in human and animal medical diagnostic laboratories: Recommendations of a CDC-convened, Biosafety Blue Ribbon Panel. *MMWR, 61*, 1–101.

Chapman, G. E. (1983). Ritual and rational action in hospitals. *Journal of Advanced Nursing, 8*, 13–20.

Cheek, J., & Gibson, T. (1996). The discursive construction of the role of the nurse in mediation administration: An exploration of the literature. *Nursing Inquiry, 3*, 83–90.

Chinn, P. (1994). A method for aesthetic knowing in nursing. In P. Chinn & J. Watson (Eds.), *Art and aesthetics in nursing* (pp. 19–40). New York, NY: National League for Nursing.

Christiansen, B. (2009). Cultivating authentic concern: Exploring how Norwegian students learn this key nursing skill. *Journal of Nursing Education, 48*, 433. doi: 10.3928/01484834-20090518-03

Clancy, T. R., Delaney, C., Morrison, B., & Gunn, J. (2006). The benefits of standardized nursing languages in complex adaptive systems such as hospitals. *Journal of Nursing Administration, 36*, 426–434.

Clarke, P. N., Watson, J., & Brewer, B. B. (2009). From theory to practice: Caring science according to Watson and Brewer. *Nursing Science Quarterly, 22*, 339–345. doi:10.1177/0894318409344769

Clarke, S. P., & Aiken, L. H. (2003). Failure to rescue. *American Journal of Nursing, 103*(1), 42–47.

Cleary, M., Walter, G., & Horsfall, J. (2009). Handover in psychiatric settings: Is change needed. *Journal of Psychosocial Nursing & Mental Health Services, 47*(3), 28–33.

Cohen, M. R., Senders, J., & Davis, N. M. (1994). Failure mode and effects analysis: A novel approach to avoiding dangerous medication errors and accidents. *Hospital Pharmacy, 29*, 324–330.

Collins, M. (2010). High impact interventions to control infection. *Emergency Nurse, 12*(10), 12–17.

Connecticut Nursing History Vignettes. Connecticut Nursing News. (n.d.). Connecticut nursing history, Eleanor Krohn Herrmann, nurse historian and professor emerita, Storrs, CT: University of Connecticut. Retrieved from http://www.legalmojo.com/article/CONNECTICUT-NURSING-HISTORY-VIGNETTES-%7C-Connecticut-Nursing-News-%7C-Find-.../1687.html

Costello, M. (2010). Changing handoffs: The shift is on. *Nursing Management, 41*(10), 39–42.

Crigger, N. J. (2004). Always having to say you're sorry: An ethical response to making mistakes in professional practice. *Nursing Ethics, 11*, 568–576. doi. 10.1191/0969733004ne739oa

Crigger, N. J., & Meek, V. L. (2007). Toward a theory of self-reconciliation following mistakes in nursing practice. *Journal of Nursing Scholarship, 39*, 177–183.

Crimlisk, J. T., Johnstone, D. J., & Sanchez, G. M. (2009). Evidence-based practice, clinical simulations workshop and intravenous medications: Moving toward safer practice. *MEDSURG Nursing, 18*, 153–160.

Davis, C. (1997). *Details of flesh*. Corvallis, OR: Calyx Books.

Davis, D. S. (1984). Good people doing dirty work: A study of social isolation. *Symbolic Interaction, 7*, 233–247.

Davis, R. (1981). The ritualization of behavior. *Mankind, 13*(2), 103–111.

Davis-Floyd, R. (1992). *Birth as an American rite of passage*. Berkeley, CA: University of California Press.

Deal, T. E., & Kennedy, A. A. (1982). *Corporate cultures: The rites and rituals of corporate life.* Reading, MA: Addison-Wesley.

DeCraemer, W., Vansina, J., & Fox, R. (1976). Religious movements in Central Africa. *Comparative Studies in Society and History, 18*, 458–475.

Dellasega, C. A. (2009). Bullying among nurses. *American Journal of Nursing, 109*(1), 52–58.

Denham, S. A. (1995). *Family routines: A construct for considering family health*. Holistic Nursing Practice, 9(4), 11–23.

Denham, S. A. (2003). Relationships between family rituals, family routines, and health. *Journal of Family Nursing, 9*, 305–330.

Dewar, A. L. (2012). Dealing with errors on the job. *Journal of Psychosocial Nursing, 50*(4), 4–5.

Dickson, G. L., & Flynn, L. (2012). Nurses' clinical reasoning: Processes and practices of medication safety. *Qualitative Health Research, 22*, 3–16. doi. 10.1177/1049732311420448. Retrieved from qhr.sagepub.com

Dictionary of the Social Sciences. Retrieved from http://dbproxy.lasalle.edu:2215/views /ENTRY.html?entry=t104.e1348&srn=1&ssid=453660720#FIRSTHIT

Douglas, M. (1966). *Purity and danger*. London, UK: Routledge & Kegan Paul.

Douglas, M. (1970). The healing rite. *Man, 5*, 302–308.

Douglas, M. (1975). *Implicit meanings: Essays in anthropology*. London, UK: Routledge & Kegan Paul.

Douglas, M. (1982). *Natural symbols: Explorations in cosmology*. New York, NY: Pantheon Books.

Douglas, M. (1999). *Implicit meanings: Selected essays in anthropology*. London, UK: Routledge.

Dowding, D. (2001). Examining the effects that manipulating information given in the change of shift report has on nurses' care planning ability. *Journal of Advanced Nursing, 33*, 836–846.

Downey, L., & Lloyd, H. (2008). Bed bathing patients in hospital. *Nursing Standard, 22*(34), 35–40.

Downs, S. H., & Black, N. (1998). The feasibility of creating a checklist for the assessment of the methodological quality both of randomised and non-randomised studies of health care interventions. *Journal of Epidemiology and Community Health, 52*, 377–384.

Drach-Zahavy, A., & Pud, D. (2010). Learning mechanisms to limit medication administration errors. *Journal of Advanced Nursing, 66*, 794–805. doi: 10.1111/j.1365-2648.2010.05294.x

Driver, T. F. (1998). *Liberating rites*. Boulder, CO: Westview.

Dunn, D. (2003). Incident reports Correcting processes and reducing errors. *AORN Journal, 78*, 212–233.

Edmonds, H. M. (1926). Baths and their uses. *Nursing Times (September 11)*, 805–806.

Eisenhauer, L. A., Hurley, A. C., & Dolan, N. (2007). Nurses' reported thinking during medication administration. *Journal of Nursing Scholarship, 39*(1), 82–87.

Ekman, I., & Segesten, K. (1995). Deputed power of medical control: The hidden message in the ritual of oral shift reports. *Journal of Advanced Nursing, 22*, 1006–1011.

Encyclopedia Judaica. (1971). *Sin* (Vol. 14). New York, NY: Macmillan.

Engebretson, J. (2002). Hands-on: The persistent metaphor in nursing. *Holistic Nursing Practice, 16*(4), 20–35.

Ergott, K. M. (2008). Hold my hand...don't let go: Moments of caring from a patient's perspective. *Journal of Holistic Nursing, 26*, 308–310.

Erickson, J. I., & Millar, S. (2005). Caring for patients while respecting their privacy: Renewing our commitment. *Online Journal of Issues in Nursing, 10*(2). Retrieved from http://nursingworld.org/MainMenuCategories/ANAMarketplace/ANAPeriodicals/OJIN/TableofContents/Volume102005/No2May05/tpc27_116017.html

Ericsson, K. A., Whyte, J., & Ward, P. (2007). Expert performance in nursing: Reviewing research on expertise in nursing within the framework of the expert-performance approach. *Advances in Nursing Science, 30*, E58–E71.

Eriksson, K. (1992). The alleviation of suffering – The idea of caring. *Scandinavian Journal of Caring Science, 6*, 119–123.

Evans, D., Grunawalt, J., McClish, D., Wood, W., & Friese, C. R. (2012). Bedside shift-to-shift nursing report: Implementation and outcomes. *MEDSURG Nursing, 21*, 281–284.

Eynan-Harvey, R. (1996). When death do us part: Nurses on post-mortem care. Master's thesis, Department of Sociology and Anthropology, Concordia University, Montréal, Québec, Canada.

Fagin, C. M., & Diers, D. (1983). Nursing ad metaphor. *New England Journal of Medicine, 309*(2), 116–117.

Fairclough, N. (1992). Discourse and text: Linguistic and intertextual analysis within discourse analysis. *Discourse and Society, 3*, 192–217.

Fallaize, K. (2007). The calmness and dignity of the last offices ritual impressed me. *Nursing Standard, 21*(38), 28.

Ferguson, K., Harvey, L., McKale-Waring, J., Platt, N., Reid, D. (2008). Pinning our hopes on the future. *Canadian Nurse, 104*(7), 9.

Finfgeld-Connett, D. (2007). Meta-synthesis of caring in nursing. *Journal of Clinical Nursing, 17*, 196–204. doi: 10.1111/j.1365-2702.2006.01824.x

Finfgeld-Connett, D. (2008a). Qualitative convergence of three nursing concepts: Art of nursing, presence and caring. *Journal of Advanced Nursing, 63*, 527–534.

Finfgeld-Connett, D. (2008b). Meta-synthesis of caring in nursing. *Journal of Clinical Nursing, 17*, 196–204.

Flora, D. S., Parsons, P. L., & Slattum, P. W. (2011). Managing medications for improved care transitions. *Generations-Journal of the American Society in Aging, 35*(4), 37–42.

Flynn, J. P., Prufeta, P. A., & Minghillo-Lipari, L. (2010). An evidence-based approach to taking charge. *American Journal of Nursing, 110*(9), 58–63.

Folkmann, L., & Rankin, J. (2010). Nurses' medication work: What do nurses know? *Journal of Clinical Nursing, 19*, 3218–3226. doi: 10.1111/j.1365-2702.2010.03249.x

Foucault, M. (1972). The archaeology of knowledge. London, UK: Routledge.

Fowler, M. D. (1984). *Ethics and nursing, 1893-1984: The ideal of service, the reality of history*. Los Angeles, CA: University of Southern California.

Free Dictionary. (n.d.). Retrieved from http://www.thefreedictionary.com/

Fredriksson, L. (1999). Modes of relating in a caring conversation: A research synthesis on presence, touch and listening. *Journal of Advanced Nursing, 30*, 1167–1176.

Fredriksson, L., & Eriksson, K. (2003). The ethics of the caring conversation. *Nursing Ethics, 10*, 138–148.

Free Dictionary. (n.d.). Retrieved from http://www.thefreedictionary.com/

Freeman, E. M. (1997). International perspectives on bathing. *Journal of Gerontological Nursing, 23*(5), 40–44.

Frost, P. J., & Wise, M. P. (2010). Managing sudden death in hospital. *British Medical Journal, 340*, c962. doi: 10.1136/bmj.c962

Fuerst, E. V., & Wolff, L. (1969). *Fundamentals of nursing* (4th ed.). Philadelphia, PA: J. B. Lippincott: Ferguson.

Gagneaux, V., & Shaver, D. V. (1977). Distractions at nurses' stations during intershift report. *Nursing Research, 26,* 42–46.

Galambos, C. (2001). Healing rituals for survivors of rape. *Advances in Social Work, 2*(1), 65–74.

Gallagher-Lepak, S., & Kubsch, S. (2009). Transpersonal caring: A nursing practice guideline. *Holistic Nursing Practice, 23,* 171–182.

Gaut, D. A. (1983). Development of a theoretically adequate description of caring. *Western Journal of Nursing Research, 5,* 313–324.

Geach, B. (1987). Bedtime ceremonials: A focus for nursing. *Archives of Psychiatric Nursing, 1,* 98–103.

Geertz, C. (1973). *The interpretation of cultures.* New York, NY: Basic Books.

Gelo, F. (1997). Risk of infection to the bereaved. *Journal of Pastoral Care, 51,* 427–430.

George, J. B. (2002). *Nursing theories: The base for professional nursing practice* (5th ed.). Upper Saddle River, NJ: Prentice Hall.

George Washington Institute for Spirituality and Health. (n.d.). FICA Spiritual History Tool. Retrieved from http://www.gwumc.edu/gwish/clinical/fica-spiritual/fica-spiritual-history/index.cfm

Gerow, L., Conejo, P., Alonzo, A., Davis, N., Rodgers, S., & Domian, E. W. (2010). Creating a curtain of protection: Nurses' experiences of grief following death. *Journal of Nursing Scholarship, 42,* 122–129.

Gilje, F. (1992). Being there: An analysis of the concept of presence. In D. A. Gaut (Ed.), *The presence of caring in nursing* (pp. 53–67). New York, NY: National League for Nursing Press.

Gilje, F. L., Klose, P. M. E., & Birger, J. (2007). Critical clinical competencies in undergraduate psychiatric-mental health nursing. *Journal of Nursing Education, 46,* 522–526.

Gill, T. M., Guo, Z., & Allore, H. G. (2006). The epidemiology of bathing disability in older persons. *Journal of the American Geriatrics Society, 54,* 1532–1530.

Ginsberg, B. (2001). Pain management in knee surgery. *Orthopedic Nursing, 20*(2), 37–44.

Gladstone, J. (1995). Drug administration errors: A study into the factors underlying the occurrence and reporting of drug errors in a district general hospital. *Journal of Advanced Nursing, 22,* 628–637.

Gluckman, M. (1975). Specificity of social-anthropological studies of ritual. *Mental Health & Society, 2,* 1–17.

Godkin, J., & Godkin, L. (2004). Caring behaviors among nurses: Fostering a conversation of gestures. *Health Care Management Review, 29,* 258–267.

Goffman, E. (1959). The presentation of self in everyday life. Garden City, NY: Doubleday.

Goffman, E. (1967). *Interaction ritual: Essays on face-to-face behavior.* New York, NY: Pantheon Books.

Goldberg, J. L. (2008). Humanism or professionalism? The white coat ceremony and medical education. *Academic Medicine: Journal of the Association of American Medical Colleges, 83,* 715–722.

Gooch, J. (1989). Skin hygiene. *Professional Nurse, 5*(1), 13, 16, 18.

Goodenough, W. H. (1964). Cultural anthropology in linguistics. In D. Hymes (Ed.), *Language in culture and society: A reader in linguistics and anthropology.* New York, NY: Harper & Row.

Grainger, M. (2011). A professional pledge would be a boost to all. *British Journal of Nursing, 20,* 477.

Grant, B. M., Giddings, L. S., & Beale, J. E. (2005). Vulnerable bodies: Competing discourses of intimate bodily care. *Journal of Nursing Education, 44,* 498-504.

Greenfield, S., Whelan, B., & Cohn, E. (2006). Use of dimensional analysis to reduce medication errors. *Journal of Nursing Education, 45,* 91–94.

Griffin, T. (2010). Bringing change-of-shift report to the bedside: A patient-and-family centered approach. *Journal of Perinatal and Neonatal Nursing, 24,* 348–353.

Grimes, R. L. (2000). *Deeply into the bone: Re-inventing rites of Passage.* Berkley, CA: University of California Press.

Groff, J. (1896). Hand-book of material medica for trained nurses. *The Trained Nurse, 16,* 635–640.

Hadders, H. (2009). Medical practice, procedure manuals and the standardization of hospital death. *Nursing Inquiry, 16*(1), 22–32.

Hales, A. (2003). Self-reflecting: Reclaiming our nursing roots. *Perspectives in Psychiatric Care, 39*(1), 5–6.

Hall, E. T. (1966). *The hidden dimension*. Garden City, NY: Anchor Books.

Halldorsdottir, S. (1991). Five basic modes of being with another. In D. Gaut & M. Leininger (Eds.), *Caring: The compassionate healer* (pp. 37–49). New York, NY: National League for Nursing.

Halldorsdottir, S. (1996). *Caring and uncaring encounters in nursing and health care. Developing a theory*. Linkoping, Sweden: Linkoping University.

Halldorsdottir, S. (2007). A psychoneuroimmunological view of healing potential of human caring in the face of human suffering. *International Journal for Human Caring, 11*(2), 32–39.

Hallett, C. E. (2010). *Celebrating nurses: A visual history*. Hauppauge, NY: Barron's.

Hammersley, M., & Atkinson, P. (1987). Feltmetodikk. Grunnlaget for feltarbeid og feltforskning. Oslo, Norway: *Gyldendal Norsk Forlag*.

Hancock, I., Bowman, A., & Prater, D. (2000). 'The day of the soft towel?' Comparison of the current bed-bathing method with the soft towel bed-bathing method. *International Journal of Nursing Practice, 6*, 207–213.

Hanrahan, N. P., Kumar, A., & Aiken, L. H. (2010). Adverse events associated with organizational factors of general hospital inpatient psychiatric care environments. *Psychiatric Services, 61*, 569–574. Retrieved from ps.psychiatryonline.org

Hansten, R., & Washburn, M. (1999). Seven steps to shift from tasks to outcomes. *Nursing Management, 3*(7), 24–27.

Happ, M. B., Tate, J. A., Swigart, V. A., DiVirgilio-Thomas, D., & Hoffman, L. A. (2010). Wash and wean: Bathing patients undergoing weaning trials during prolonged mechanical ventilation. *Heart & Lung, 39*(6S), S47–S56.

Hardey, M., Payne, S., & Coleman, P. (2000). 'Scraps': Hidden nursing information and its influence on the delivery of care. *Journal of Advanced Nursing, 32*, 208–214.

Harding, L., & Petrick, T. (2008). Nursing student medication errors: A retrospective review. *Journal of Nursing Education, 47*(1), 43–47.

Hardy, M. A. (1990). A pilot study of the diagnosis and treatment of impaired skin integrity: Dry skin in older persons. *Nursing Diagnosis, 1*(2), 57–63.

Harrison, L., & Nixon, G. (2002). Nursing activity in general intensive care. *Journal of Clinical Nursing, 11*, 158–167. See p. 159 for hidden work paraphrase.

Hartig, M. T. (1998). Expert nursing assistant care activities. *Western Journal of Nursing Research, 20*, 584–601.

Hartwig, S. C., Denger, S. D., & Schneider, P. J. (1991). A severity-indexed, incident report-based medication-error reporting program. *American Journal of Hospital Pharmacy, 48*, 2611–2612.

Hawkins, P., & Redding, S. R. (2004). Commissioning ceremony. *Nurse Educator, 29*, 133–134.

Hawknurse. (2008). Giving a patient a bed bath. *YouTube*. Retrieved from http://www.youtube.com/watch?v-hYXYcOHT6aE

Hayes, K. (2005). Designing written medication instructions: Effective ways to help older adults self-medicate. *Journal of Gerontological Nursing, 31*(5), 5–47. Retrieved from ProQuest Central.

Hays, M. M. (2003). The phenomenal shift report. *Journal for Nurses in Staff Development, 19*, 25–33.

Hays, M. M., & Weinert, C. (2006). A dramaturgical analysis of shift report patterns with cost implications: A case study. *Nursing Economics, 24*, 253–262.

Hektor, L. M., & Touhy, T. A. (1997). The history of the bath: From art to task? Reflections on the future. *Journal of Gerontological Nursing, 23*(5), 7–15.

Heliker, D., & Scholler-Jaquish, A. (2006). Transition of new residents: Basing practice on residents' perspective. *Journal of Gerontological Nursing*, September, 34–42.

Helman, G. C. (1990). Culture, health and illness. Oxford, UK: Butterworth Heinemann.

Henricson, M., Segesten, K., Berglund, A-L., & Määtä, S. (2009). Enjoying tactile touch and gaining hope when being cared for in intensive care A phenomenological hermeneutical study. *Intensive and Critical Care Nursing, 25*, 323–331.

Hertzel, C., & Sousa, V. D. (2009). The use of smart pumps for preventing medication errors. *Journal of Infusion Nursing, 32,* 257–267.

Higgins, D. (2008a). Carrying out last offices: Part 1-preparing for the procedure. *Nursing Times, 104*(37), 20–21.

Higgins, D. (2008b). Carrying out last offices: Part 2-preparation of the body. *Nursing Times, 104*(38), 24–25.

Hills, M., & Albarran, J. W. (2010a). After death 1: Caring for bereaved relatives and being aware of cultural differences. *Nursing Times, 106*(27), 19–20.

Hills, M., & Albarran, J. W. (2010b). After death 2: Exploring the procedures for laying out and preparing the body for viewing. *Nursing Times, 106*(28), 22–24.

Hodo, A., & Buller, L. (2012). Managing care at the end of life. *Nursing Management, 48*(3), 28–33.

Holden, J. (2006). Just follow your nose. *Nursing Standard, 20*(41), 30–31.

Holland, C. K. (1993). An ethnographic study of nursing culture as an exploration for determining the existence of a system of ritual. *Journal of Advanced Nursing, 18,* 1461–1470.

Holmes, D., Perron, A., & O'Byrne, P. (2006). Understanding disgust in nursing: Abjection, self, and the other. *Research and Theory for Nursing Practice: An International Journal, 20,* 305–315.

Holmes Regional Medical Center and Palm Bay Community Hospital. (2006). Nursing management's Visionary Leader 2005: Elizabeth Manco-Herrman. *Nursing Management, 37*(1), 20–22.

Hopkinson, J. (2002). The hidden benefit: The supportive function of the nursing handover for qualified nursing caring for dying people in hospital. *Journal of Clinical Nursing, 11,* 168–175.

Huber, S. J. (2003). The white coat ceremony: A contemporary medical ritual. *Journal of Medical Ethics, 29,* 364–366.

Hudson, K. (2009, September 28). Safe medication administration. Retrieved from http://dynamicnursingeducation.com/class.php?class_id=38&pid=15

Huey, F. L. (1986). Working smart. *American Journal of Nursing, 86,* 679–684.

Huttmann, B. (1985). Quit wasting time with "nursing rituals." *Nursing, 15,* 34–39.

Institute for Safe Medication Practices (ISMP). (2004). The five rights cannot stand alone. *Nurse Advise-ERR, 2*(11), 1–2. Retrieved from http://www.ismp.org/Newsletters/nursing/Issues/NurseAdviseERR200411.pdf

Institute for Safe Medication Practices (ISMP). (2007, January 25). The five rights: A destination without a map. ISMP medication Safety Alert! Retrieved from http://www.ismp.org/newsletters/acutecare/articles/20070125.asp

Jarrin, O. F. (2006). Results from the Nurse Manifest 2003 Study: Nurses' perspectives on nursing. *Advances in Nursing Science, 29,* E74–E85.

Jasovsky, D. A., Grant, V. A., Lang, M., Devereux, B. F., Altier, M. E., Bird, S. R., … Hindle, P. A. (2010). How do you define nursing excellence? *Nursing Management, 41*(10), 19–24.

Jeffries, P. R., Rew, R., & Cramer, J. M. (2002). A comparison of student-centered versus traditional methods of teaching basic nursing skills in a learning laboratory. *Nursing Education Perspectives, 23*(1), 14–19.

Jennings, B. M., Sandelowski, M., & Mark, B. (2011). The nurse's medication day. *Qualitative Health Research, 21,* 1441–1451. Retrieved from qhr.sagepub.com

Jervis, L. I. (2001). The pollution of incontinence and the dirty work of caregiving in a U.S. nursing home. *Medical Anthropology Quarterly, 15*(1), 84–99.

Jha, A. K., Desroches, C. M., Campbell, E. G., Donelan, K., Rao, S. R., Ferris, T. G., et al. (2009). The use of electronic health records in U.S. hospitals. *New England Journal of Medicine, 360,* 1628–1638.

Johanna Briggs Institute. (2006). Strategies to reduce medication errors with reference to older adults. *Nursing Standard, 20*(41), 53–57.

Johnson, J. L. (1994). A dialectical examination of nursing art. *Advances in Nursing Sciences, 17*(1), 1–14.

Johansson, I. M., Skärsäter, I., & Danielson, E. (2007). Encounters in a locked psychiatric ward environment. *Journal of Psychiatric and Mental Health Nursing, 14*, 366–372.

John Dempsey Hospital. (2012, March). Post mortem care. *Clinical Procedure, Clinical Manual/ Nursing Practice Manual*, 1–5. Retrieved from http://nursing.uchc.edu/nursing_standards /docs/Post%20Mortem%20Care.pdf

Johnson, M., & Young, H. (2011). The application of Aronson's taxonomy to medication errors in nursing. *Journal of Nursing Care Quality, 26*, 128–135.

The Joint Commission. (2009, April 1). Affirmation statement. Retrieved from http://www .jointcommission.org/Affirmation_Statement

The Joint Commission. Sentinel events. Retrieved at http://www.jointcommission.org /topics/hai_sentinel_event.aspx

The Joint Commission. (2010). Sentinel event data event type by year: 195-fourth quarter 2010. Chicago, IL: Author. Retrieved from http://www.jointcommission.org/sentinel _event_data_general/

The Joint Commission. (2011, January 4). Sentinel event policy and procedures. Retrieved from http://www.jointcommission.org/Sentinel_Event_Policy_and_Procedures

Jones, A. H. (1988). *Images of nurses: Perspectives from history, art, and literature*. Philadelphia, PA: University of Pennsylvania Press.

Jost, S. G., & Rich, V. L. (2010). Transformation of a nursing culture through actualization of a nursing professional practice model. *Nursing Administration Quarterly, 34*(1), 30–40.

Jourard, S. (1971). The transparent self. New York, NY: D. Van Nostrand.

Jowett, R. (1997). Declaration of good character. What does this mean? *Journal of Clinical Nursing, 6*, 83–84.

Jukkala, A. M., James, D., Autrey, P., & Azuero, A. (2012). Developing a standardized tool to improve nurse communication during shift report. *Journal of Nursing Care Quality, 27*, 240–246.

Jury, L. A., Gierrero, D. M., Burant, C. J., Cadnum, J. L., & Donskey, C. J. (2011). Effectiveness of routine patient bathing to decrease the burden of sores on the skin of patients with *Clostridium difficile* infection. *Infection Control and Hospital Epidemiology, 32*, 180–184.

Kafka, J. S. (1983). Challenge and confirmation in ritual action. *Psychiatry, 46*, 31–39.

Kalisch, B. J., Begeny, S., & Anderson, C. (2008). The effect of consistent nursing shifts on teamwork and continuity of care. *Journal of Nursing Administration, 38*, 132–137.

Kansas State Nurses Association. (2012). The Nightingale Ceremony. Retrieved from http: //www.ksnurses.com/the-nightingale-tribute.html

Keating, J. (2009). Care after death. *Nursing Standard, 23*(26), 59.

Kent, H., & McDowell, J. (2004). Sudden bereavement in acute care setting. *Nursing Standard, 19*(6), 38–42.

Kerr, M. P. (2002). A qualitative study of shift handover practice and function from a socio-technical perspective. *Journal of Advanced Nursing, 37*, 125–134.

King, I. (1996). Theory of goal attainment in research and practice. *Nursing Science Quarterly, 9*(2), 61–66.

Kongsuwan, W., & Locsin, R. C. (2011). Thai nurses' experience of caring for person with life-sustaining technologies in intensive care settings: A phenomenological study. *Intensive and Critical Care Nursing, 27*, 102–110.

Kovach, C. R., & Meyer-Arnold, E. A. (1996). Coping with conflicting agendas: The bathing experience of cognitively impaired older adults. *Scholarly Inquiry for Nursing Practice: An International Journal, 10*(1), 23–36.

Kozier, B., Erb, G., & Olivieri, R. (Eds.). (1991). *Fundamentals of nursing: Concepts, process, and practice* (4th ed.). Redwood City, CA: Addison-Wesley.

Krippendorff, K. (2004). Content analysis: An introduction to its methodology (2nd ed.). Thousand Oaks, CA: Sage.

Kwan, C. (2002). Families' experiences of the last office of deceased family members in the hospice setting. *International Journal of Palliative Nursing, 8*, 266–275.

Lakomy, J. M. (1994). Healing rituals experienced by persons living with AIDS. In D. A. Gaut, & A. Boykin (Eds.), *Caring as healing: Renewal through hope* (pp. 241–251). New York, NY: National League for Nursing Press.

Lamond, D. (2000). The information content of the nurse change of shift report: A comparative study. *Journal of Advanced Nursing, 31*, 794–804.

Larson, E. L., Ciliberti, T., Chantler, C., Abraham, J., Lazaro, E. M., Venturanza, M., & Pancholi, P. Comparison of traditional and disposable bed baths in critically ill patients. *American Journal of Critical Care, 13*, 235–241.

Lavery, I. (2011). Intravenous therapy: Preparation and administration of IV medicines. *British Journal of Nursing, 20*(4), S28–S34.

Lawler, J. (1991). *Behind the screens: Nursing, somology, and the problem of the body*. Melbourne, Australia: Churchill Livingstone.

Lee, C. J., Idczak, S., Moon, J., & Brown-Schott, N. (2006). Strong minds, healing hands, and compassionate hearts: Developing a contemporary and creative twist on tradition. *Nursing Education Perspectives, 27*(11), 10–11.

Legare, C. H., & Souza, A. L. (2012). Evaluating ritual efficacy: Evidence from the supernatural. *Cognition, 124*, 1–15.

LeMaire, B. (2002, March 15). Eleanor Herrmann, on the history of nursing. Retrieved from http://www.nurseweek.com/5min/herrmann.asp

Leuba, J. H. (1909). Magic and religion. *Sociologic Review, a2*(1), 20–35.

Lim, F. A. (2011). Questioning: A teaching strategy to foster clinical thinking and reasoning. *Nurse Educator, 36*, 52–53.

Lindseth, A., & Norberg, A. (2004). A phenomenological hermeneutical method for researching lived experience. *Scandinavian Journal of Caring Sciences, 18*, 145–153.

Lohman, E. L. (1933). Pouring and passing medicine. *American Journal of Nursing, 33*(1), 29–31.

Lomborg, K., Bjørn, A., Dahl, R., Kirkevold, M. (2005). Body care experiences by people hospitalized with severe respiratory disease. *Journal of Advanced Nursing, 50*, 262–271.

Lomborg, K., & Kirkevold, M. (2005). Curtailing: Handling the complexity of body care in people hospitalized with severe COPD. *Scandinavian Journal of Caring Sciences, 19*, 148–156.

Lomborg, K., & Kirkevold, M. (2008). Achieving therapeutic clarity in assisted personal body care: Professional challenges in interactions with severely ill COPD patients. *Journal of Clinical Nursing, 17*(16), 2155–2163. doi: 10.1111/j.1365-2702.2006.01710.x

Lundberg, K. M. (2008). Promoting self-confidence in clinical nursing students. *Nurse Educator, 33*, 86–89.

Lynch, M., & Dahlin, C. M. (2007). The National Consensus Project and National Quality Forum preferred practices in care of the imminently dying. *Journal of Hospice and Palliative Nursing, 9*, 316–322.

MacDavitt, K., Cieplinski, J. A., & Walker, V. (2011). Implementing small tests of change to improve patient satisfaction. *Journal of Nursing Administration, 41*, 5–9.

Macleod, M. (1994). "It's the little things that count": The hidden complexity of everyday clinical nursing practice. *Journal of Clinical Nursing, 3*, 361–368.

Madsen, W., McAllister, M., Godden, J., Greenhill, J., & Reed, R. (2009). Nursing orphans: How the system of nursing education in Australia is undermining professional identity. *Contemporary Nurse, 32*(1–2), 9–18.

Mahoney, E. K., Trudeau, S. A., Penyack, S. E., & MacLeod, C. E. (2006). Challenges to intervention implementation: Lessons learned in the bathing persons with Alzheimer's Disease at home study. *Nursing Research, 55*(2S), S10–S16.

Malinowski, B. (1954). *Magic, science, and religion and other essays*. Garden City, NY: Rand McNally.

Malinowski, B. (1992). *Magic, science and religion and other essays*. Prospect Heights, IL: Waveland Press.

Mandrack, M., Cohen, M. R., Featherling, J., Gellner, L., Judd, K., Kienle, P. C., & Vanderveen, T. (2012). Nursing best practices using automated dispensing cabinets: Nurses' key role in improving medication safety. *MEDSURG Nursing, 21*, 134–144.

Manias, E., & Street, A. (2000). The handover: Uncovering the hidden practices of nurses. *Intensive and Critical Care Nursing, 16*, 373–383.

Manning, M. L. (2006). Improving clinical communication through structured conversation. *Nursing Economics, 24*, 268–271.

Maricle, K., Whitehead, L., & Rhodes, M. (2007). Examining medication errors in a tertiary hospital. *Journal of Nursing Care Quality, 22*(1), 20–27.

Martin, G. (1998). Ritual action and its effect on the role of the nurse as advocate. *Journal of Advanced Nursing, 27*, 189–194.

Martinsen, K. (1997). Fra Marx til Logstrup: Om etikk og sanselighet i sykepleien. Oslo, Norway, Tano.

Martinsen, K. (2000). Oyet og kallet. Bergen, Norway: Fagbokforlaget Vigmostad og Bjorke.

Mason, D. J. (2004). Shift to shift. *American Journal of Nursing, 104*(9), 11.

Matic, J., Davidson, P. M., & Salamonson, Y. (2010). Review: Bring patient safety to the forefront through structured computerization during clinical handover. *Journal of Clinical Nursing, 20*, 184–189.

Matzo, M. L. (2004). Peri-death nursing care. In M. L. Matzo & D. W. Sherman, *Gerontologic palliative care nursing* (pp. 499–533). St. Louis, MO: Mosby.

Maxson, P. M., Derby, K. M., Wrobleski, D. M., & Foss, D. M. (2012). Bedside nurse-to-nurse handoff promotes patient safety. *MEDSURG Nursing, 21*, 140–145.

Mayring, P. (1997). Qualitative inhaltsanalyse: Grundlagen und techniken. 6, durchges. Dt. Studien-Verl, Weinheim.

McAllister, M., John, T., & Gray, M. (2009). In my day: Using lessons from history, ritual and our elders to build professional identity. *Nurse Education in Practice, 9*, 277–283.

McBurney, B. H., & Filoromo, T. (1994). The Nightingale Pledge: 100 years later. *Nursing Management, 25*(2), 72–74.

McCloughen, A., O'Brien, L., Gillies, D., & McSherry, C. (2008). Nursing handover within mental health rehabilitation: An exploratory study of practice and perception. *International Journal of Mental Health Nursing, 17*, 287–295. doi: 10.1111/j.1447-0349.2008.00545.x

McCreery, J. (1979). Potential and effective meaning in therapeutic ritual. *Culture, Medicine and Psychiatry, 3*, 53–72.

McGraw, C., & Drennan, V. (2009). Assisting older people with bathing. *Journal of Community Nursing, 23*(9), 12–16.

McGuigan, D., & Gilbert, S. (2009). An educational programme for end of life care in an acute care setting. *Nursing Standard, 23*(49), 35–40.

Mehta, K. M., Pierluissi, E., Boscardin, J., Kirby, K. A., Walter, L. C., Chren, M-M., … Landefeld, C. S. (2011). A clinical index to stratify hospitalized older adults according to risk for new-onset disability. *Journal of the American Geriatrics Society, 59*, 1206–1216.

Mellichamp, P. (2007). End-of-life care for infants. *Home Healthcare Nurse, 25*(1), 41–44.

Merriam-Webster. (n.d.). Retrieved from http://www.merriam-webster.com/

Merton, R. K. (1968). *Social theory and social structure* (rev. ed.). New York, NY: Free Press.

Meyer, G., & Lavin, M. A. (2005). Vigilance: The essence of nursing. *Online Journal of Issues in Nursing, 10*(3), 8. Retrieved from http://www.nursingworld.org/MainMenuCategories/ANAMarketplace/ANAPeriodicals/OJIN/TableofContents/Volume102005/No3Sept05/ArticlePreviousTopic/VigilanceTheEssenceofNursing.aspx

Miller, E. T. (2011). Medication safety: An essential nursing role. *Rehabilitation Nursing, 38*, 134, 174.

Miller, G. A. (1956). The magical number seven, plus or minus two: Some limits on our capacity for processing information. *Psychological Review, 63*, 81–97.

Miller-Keane, M. (2003). *Miller–Keane encyclopedia and dictionary of medicine, nursing, and allied health* (7th ed.). Philadelphia, PA: Saunders/Elsevier.

Millner, P., Paskiewicz, S. T., & Kautz, D. (2009). A comfortable place to say goodbye. *Dimensions of Critical Care Nursing, 28*(1), 13–17.

Morse, J. M., Bottorff, J., Anderson, G., O'Brien, B., & Solberg, S. (1992). Beyond empathy: Expanding expressions of caring. *Journal of Advanced Nursing, 17*, 809–821.

Morse, J. M., Bottorff, J., Neander, W., & Solberg, S. (1991). Comparative analysis of conceptualizations and theories of caring. Image: *Journal of Nursing Scholarship, 23*, 119–126.

Mosher, C., & Bontomasi, R. (1996). How to improve your shift report. *American Journal of Nursing, 96*(8), 32–34.

Muir, N. (2002). Dealing with death. *Nursing Standard, 17*(3), 33.

Mulhall, A. (1996). The cultural context of death: What nurses need to know. *Nursing Times, 92*(34), 38–40.

Mungall, D. (2008). Honour of carrying out last offices helped calm my nerves. *Nursing Standard, 22*(46), 29.

Munhall, P. (Ed.). (2007). *Nursing research: A qualitative perspective* (4th ed.). Sudbury, MA: Jones & Bartlett.

Munn, N. D. (1973). Symbolism in a ritual context: Aspects of symbolic action. In J. Honigmann (Ed.), *Handbook of social and cultural anthropology* (pp. 579–611). Chicago, IL: Rand McNally.

Murdock, G. P., Ford, C. S., Hudson, A. E., Kennedy, R., Simmons, L. W., & Whiting, J. W. M. (1961). *Outline of cultural materials* (Vol. 1, 4th rev. ed.). New Haven, CT: Human Relations Area Files.

Murray, K. (2009). Implementing change. Male nurses in labor and delivery: bedside shift report. *Nursing Management, 40*(10), 56.

Myers, H. R. (n.d.). How to perform post-mortem care. Retrieved from www.ehow.com/how_4811191_perform-postmortem-care.html

Nåden, D., & Eriksson, K. (2000). The phenomenon of confirmation: An aspect of nursing as an art. *International Journal for Human Caring, 4*(2), 23–28.

National Coordinating Council for Medication Error Reporting and Prevention (NCC MERP). (2001). NCC MERP Index for categorizing medication errors. Retrieved from http://www.nccmerp.org/pdf/indexColor2001-06-12.pdf

National Coordinating Council for Medication Error Reporting and Prevention (NCC MERP). (2012). What is a medication error? Retrieved from http://www.nccmerp.org/aboutMedErrors.html?USP_Print=true&frame=lowerfrm

National League for Nursing (NLN). (n.d.). Academy of nursing education. Retrieved from http://www.nln.org/excellence/academy/index.htm

Nelson, B. A., & Massey, R. (2010). Implementing an electronic change-of-shift report using transforming care at the bedside processes and methods. *Journal of Nursing Administration, 40*, 162–168.

Newell, A., & Simon, H. A. (1972). Human problem solving. Upper Saddle River, NJ: Prentice-Hall.

Newland, J. A. (2011). National Nurses Week: A time for reflection and celebration. *Nurse Practitioner, 36*(5), 5.

New York City Health and Hospitals Corporation. (n.d.). HHC about Bellevue. Retrieved from http://www.nyc.gov/html/hhc/bellevue/html/about/history.shtml

Nicholas, P. K., & Agius, C. R. (2005). Toward safer IV medication administration. *American Journal of Nursing, 102*(Suppl 3), 25–30.

Nguyen, E. R., Connolly, P. M., & Wong, V. (2010). Medication safety initiative in reducing medication errors. *Journal of Nursing Care Quality, 25*, 224–230.

Nursing2012 Drug Handbook. (2012). Philadelphia, PA: Lippincott Williams & Wilkins. Retrieved from http://www.nursingcenter.com/Blog/category/Medication-errors.aspx

Nursing Connection. The origin of nursing school pins. Retrieved from http://www.kbn .gov/NR/rdonlytes/A0C03F9F-868F-4EB3-8905-20FAA18F2445/0/KBN

Nursing Student. (2008). Seeing a dead body helped me deal with my mother's illness. *Nursing Standard, 22*(42), 26.

Nyatanga, B., & de Vocht, H. (2009). When last offices are more than just a white sheet. *British Journal of Nursing, 18,* 1028.

Ocean County College. (2008). Pinning ceremony. Retrieved from http://www.ocean.edu /academics/programs_of_study/nursing/pinningceremony.htm

O'Horo, J. C., Silva, G. L., Munoz-Price, S., & Safdar, N. (2012). The efficacy of daily bathing with chlorhexidine for reducing healthcare-associate bloodstream infections: A meta-analysis. *Infection Control and Hospital Epidemiology, 33,* 257–267.

O'Regan, H., & Fawcett, T. (2006). Learning to nurse: Reflections on bathing a patient. *Nursing Standard, 20*(46), 60–64.

Ott, B. B., Al-Junaibi, S., & Al-Khaduri, J. (2003). Preventing ethical dilemmas: Understanding Islamic health care practices. *Pediatric Nursing, 29,* 227–230.

Pacis, C. R. (1986). A comparison of three methods of temperature control. *Academy of Nursing in the Philippines, 21*(2), 20–28.

Padilha, M. I., & Nelson, S. (2011). Networks of identity: The potential of biographical studies for teaching nursing identity. *Nursing History Review, 19,* 183–193. doi: http://dx.doi .org/10.1891/1062-8061.19.183

Padmanabhan, M. (2003). XVII lamp lighting ceremony 2003. *Nursing Journal of India, 94*(5), 111.

Parker, M. E. (1993). *Patterns of nursing theories in practice.* New York, NY: National League for Nursing Press.

Parsons, C. L., Peard, A. L., & Page, C. (1985). The effects of hygiene interventions on the cerebrovascular status of severe closed head injured persons. *Research in Nursing and Health, 8,* 173–181.

Pasquale, P. (2008). Reclaiming our "nursing fundamentals": Don't comfort and hygiene matter any more? *American Journal of Nursing, 108*(10), 11.

Paterson, J., & Zderad, L. T. (1976). *Humanistic Nursing.* New York, NY: John Wiley & Sons, Inc.

Paterson, J. G., & Zderad, L. T. (1998). *Humanistic Nursing.* New York, NY: National League for Nursing.

Paterson, B. L. (2001). The shifting perspectives model of chronic illness. Image: *Journal of Nursing Scholarship, 33,* 21–26.

Pattison, N. (2007). Caring for patients after death. *Nursing Standard, 22*(51), 48–56.

Payne, S., Hardey, M., & Coleman, P. (2000). Interactions between nurses during handovers in elderly care. *Journal of Advanced Nursing, 32,* 277–285.

Peltier, B. N. (2004). White coat principles. *Journal of the American College of Dentists, 71*(4), 53–56.

Pennington, E. A. (1978). Postmortem care: More than ritual. *American Journal of Nursing, 78,* 846–847.

Peplau, H. (1952). *Interpersonal relations in nursing.* New York, NY: Springer.

Peplau, H. (1992). *Interpersonal relations in nursing.* London, UK: Macmillan.

Perry, B. (2002). Grow and satisfaction: "I became a nurse because I want to help others" is a common response when people are asked why they entered nursing. As this researcher found, it is in the many ways of meeting this desire that nurses reach their highest goal. *Canadian Nurse, 98*(10), 19–22.

Philpin, S. M. (2002). Rituals and nursing: A critical commentary. *Journal of Advanced Nursing, 38,* 144–151.

Picco, E., Santoro, R., & Garrino, L. (2010). Dealing with the patient's body in nursing: Nurses' ambiguous experience in clinical practice. *Nursing Inquiry, 17*(1), 38–45.

Pinkerton, S. E. (2003). Mentoring new graduates. *Nursing Economics, 21,* 202–203.

Pipe, T. B., Connolly, T., Spahr, N., Lendzion, N., Buchda, V., Jury, R., & Cisar, N. (2012). Bringing back the basics of nursing: Defining patient care essentials. *Nursing Administration Quarterly, 36*, 225–233.

Post, K., & Righi, S. (2010). Helping nurses SHINE. *Nursing Management, 41*(11), 8–13.

Pothier, D., Monteiro, P., Mooktiar, M., & Shaw, A. (2005). Pilot student to show the loss of important data in nursing handover. *British Journal of Nursing, 14*, 1090–1093.

Potter, P., Boxerman, S., Wolf, L., Marshall, J., Grayson, D., Sledge, J., & Evanoff, B. (2004). Mapping the nursing process: A new approach for understanding the work of nursing. *Journal of Nursing Administration, 34*, 101–109.

Potter, P. A. & Perry, A. G. (2003). *Basic nursing: Essentials for practice* (5th ed.). St. Louis, MO: Mosby.

Potter, P., Sledge, J., Wolf, L., Dunagan, S., Boxerma, S., Evanoff, B., & Grayson, D. (2005). Understanding the cognitive work of nursing in the acute care environment. *Journal of Nursing Administration, 35*, 327–335.

Preston, M. (2011). Watching a child die taught me that not everyone can be helped. *Nursing Standard, 25*(42), 27.

Pulchaski, C. M. (2006). *A time for listening and caring: Spirituality and the care of the chronically ill and dying.* New York, NY: Oxford University Press.

Quested, B., & Rudge, T. (2003). Nursing care of dead bodies: A discursive analysis of last offices. *Journal of Advanced Nursing, 41*, 553–560.

Quinn, J. F. (1992). Holding sacred space: The nurse as healing environment. *Holistic Nursing Practice, 6*(4), 26–36.

Quinlan, K. (1999). A father helps with postmortem care. *Journal of Emergency Nursing, 25*, 353.

Rader, J., Barrick, A. L., Hoeffer, B., Sloane, P. D., McKenzie, D., Talerico, K. A., & Glover, J. U. (2006). The bathing of older adults with dementia. *American Journal of Nursing, 104*(4), 40–48.

Råholm, M-B., & Lindholm, L. (1999). Being in the world of the suffering patient: A challenge to nursing ethics. *Nursing Ethics, 6*, 528–539.

Ranheim, A., Kärner, A., & Berterö, C. (2012). Caring theory and practice—Entering a simultaneous concept analysis. *Nursing Forum, 47*(2), 78–90.

Reason, J. (1990). *Human error.* Cambridge, United Kingdom: Cambridge University Press.

Reason, J. (1995). Understanding adverse events: Human factors. *Quality in Health Care, 4*, 80–89.

Reason, J. (2000). Human error: Models and management. *British Medical Journal, 320*, 768–770.

Reed, M. M. (2009, August 5). *American nursing pins in history and in context. Nursing school graduation pins and collectibles.* Retrieved from https://sites.google.com/site/nursing pinsandcollectibles

Reid, M., McDowell, J., & Hoskins, R. (2011). Breaking news of death to relatives. *Nursing Times, 107*(5), 12–15.

Reid-Searl, K., & Happell, B. (2012). Supervising nursing students administering medication: A perspective from registered nurses. *Journal of Clinical Nursing, 21*, 1998–2005. doi: 10.1111/j.1365-2702.2011.03976.x

Renouf, J. (2012). Sitting in silence with grieving parents gave them support. *Nursing Standard, 26*(36), 29.

Richard, J. A. (1988). Congruence between intershift reports and patients' actual conditions. *Image: Journal of Nursing Scholarship, 20*, 4–6.

Ricoeur, P. (1992). Oneself as another. Chicago, IL: University of Chicago Press.

Riesenberg, L. A., Leitzsch, J., & Cunningham, J. M. (2010). Nursing handoffs: A systematic review of the literature. *American Journal of Nursing, 110*(4), 24–34.

Roach, M. S. (2002). *Caring: The human mode of being.* Ottawa, Ontario: CHA Press.

Robert Wood Johnson Foundation. (2008, May 15). *Introducing interdisciplinary palliative care services in seven intensive care units.* Seattle, WA: University of Washington. Grant ID# 047996.

Robichaud-Ekstrand, S. (1991). Shower versus sink bath: Evaluation of heart rate, blood pressure, and subjective response of the patient with myocardial infarction. *Heart & Lung, 20,* 375–382.

Rode, M. W. (1989). The nursing pin: Symbol of 1,000 years of service. *Nursing Forum, 24*(1), 15–17.

Rosenberg, C. E. (1987). *The care of strangers: The rise of America's hospital system.* New York, NY: Basic Books.

Rosenthal, K. (2004). Smart pumps help crack the safety code. *Nursing Management, 35*(5), 49–51.

Routasalo, P. (1999). Physical touch in nursing studies. *Journal of Advanced Nursing, 30,* 843–850.

Royal Commission for Long Term Care. (1999). Independent Review of Free Personal and Nursing Care in Scotland. Retrieved from http://www.scotland.gov.uk/Publications/2008/04/25105036/5

Rozzini, R., Sabatini, T., Ranhoff, A. H., & Trabucchi, M. (2007). Bathing disability in older patients. *Journal of the American Geriatrics Society, 55,* 635.

Ruland, C. M., & Moore, S. M. (1998). Theory construction based on standards of care: A proposed theory of the peaceful end of life. *Nursing Outlook, 46,* 169–175.

Rushton, C. H. (2010). Ethics of nursing shift report. *AACN Advanced Critical Care, 21,* 380–383.

Sanghera, I. S., Franklin, B. D., & Dhillon, S. (2007). The attitudes and beliefs of healthcare professionals on the causes and reporting of medication errors in a UK intensive care unit. *Anaesthesia, 62,* 53–61. doi: 10.1111/j.1365-2044.2006.04858.x

Sankar, A. (1991). Ritual and dying: A cultural analysis of social support for caregivers. *Gerontologist, 31*(1), 43–50.

Savage, J. (1997). Gestures of resistance: The nurse's body in contested space. *Nursing Inquiry, 4,* 237–245.

Scalise, D. (2006). Clinical communication and patient safety. Retrieved from http://www.hhnmag.com/hhnmag/jsp/articledisplay.jsp?dcrpath=HHNMAG/PubsNewsArticle/data/2006August/0608HHN_gatefold&domain=HHNMAG

Scanlon, N. (2005). Ending the paper chase. *Nursing Management, 11*(10), 24–27.

Schmahl, J. A. (1964). Ritualism in nursing practice. *Nursing Forum, 3*(4), 74–84.

Scott, H. (2004). Are nurses "too clever to care" or "too posh to wash?" *British Journal of Nursing, 13,* 581.

Scovell, S. (2010). Role of the nurse-to-nurse handover in patient care. *Nursing Standard, 24*(20), 35–39.

Sexton, A., Chan, C., Elliott, M., Stuart, J., Jayasuriya, R., & Crookes, P. (2004). Nursing handovers: Do we *really* need them? *Journal of Nursing Management, 12,* 37–42.

Shakespeare, P. (2003). Nurses' bodywork: Is there a body of work? *Nursing Inquiry, 10*(1), 47–56.

Sharoff, L. (2009). Expressiveness and creativeness: Metaphorical images of nursing. *Nursing Science Quarterly, 22,* 312–317.

Shaw, M. J. (2003). Correct administration of topical eye treatment. *Nursing Standard, 17*(30), 42–44.

Shaw, I. (2004). Doctors, "dirty work" patients, and "revolving doors." *Qualitative Health Research, 14,* 1032–1045. doi: 10.1177/1049732304265928

Sheldon, N. S. (1953). Bathing the patient. *American Journal of Nursing, 53,* 1451–1454.

Sherman, A., & Mitty, E. (2008). Transforming personal care through ritual. *Geriatric Nursing, 29,* 412–420.

Sieger, M., Fritz, E., & Them, C. (2011). In discourse: Bourdieu's theory of practice and habitus in the context of a communication-oriented nursing interaction model. *Journal of Advanced Nursing, 68,* 480–489. doi: 10.1111/j.1365–2648.2011.05783.x

Sims, C. E. (2003). Increasing clinical, satisfaction and financial performance through nurse-driven process improvement. *Journal of Nursing Administration, 33,* 68–75.

Skaalvik, M. W., Normann, H. K., & Henriksen, N. (2010). To what extent does the oral shift report stimulate learning among nursing students? A qualitative study. *Journal of Clinical Nursing, 19,* 2300–2308.

Skewes, S. (1994). No more bed baths! *RN, 57*(1), 34–35.

Skewes, S. M. (1996). Skin care rituals that do more harm than good. *American Journal of Nursing, 96*(10), 33–35.

Skillman-Hull, L. E. (1994). *She walks in beauty: Nurse-artists' lived experience of the creative process and aesthetic human care.* School of Nursing, University of Colorado. (UMI # 9426105).

Skultans, V. (1980, June). A dying ritual. *Mims Magazine,* 43–47.

Smeltzer, S. C., Bare, B. G., Hinkle, J. L., & Cheever, K. H. (2008). *Brunner & Suddarth's textbook of medical-surgical nursing* (11th ed.). Philadelphia, PA: Lippincott Williams & Wilkins.

Smith, A. C. T., & Stewart, B. (2010). Organizational rituals: Features, functions and mechanisms. *International Journal of Management Reviews, 13,* 113–133.

Smith, E. L. (2003). Making the Magnet commitment. *Journal for Nurses in Staff Development, 19,* 272–276.

Smith, M. E. (1900a). Baths and bathing. *The Trained Nurse and Hospital Review, 25*(1), 18–22.

Smith, M. E. (1900b). Baths and bathing. *The Trained Nurse and Hospital Review, 25*(2), 97–101.

Smith, O. K. (1936). Therapeutic temperature bath in childhood syphilis. *American Journal of Nursing, 36,* 693–696.

Smith, R., Snedeker, L., Rivera, K., Willier, T., & Mortimer, M. L. (2012). NICU bath basin study: Basins with growth (abstract). *American Journal of Infection Control, 40,* e152–e153.

Smith-Stoner, M., & Hand, M. W. (2012). Expanding the concept of patient care: Analysis of postmortem policies in California hospitals. *MEDSURG Nursing, 21,* 360–366.

Snow, A. F., & Bozeman, J. M. (2010). Role implications for nurses caring for gunshot wound victims. *Critical Care Nursing Quarterly, 33,* 259–264.

Speas, J. (2004). A shift in staff relationships. *Holistic Nursing Practice, 18,* 235–237.

Speas, J. (2006). Bolster staff relations with shift report. *Nursing Management, 37*(10), 82–83.

Speck, P. (1992). Care after death…cleansing and shrouding the body. *Nursing Times, 88*(6), 5–11.

Spradley, J. (1979). The ethnographic interview. New York, NY: Holt, Rinehart & Winston.

Stackpoole, F. (1889). Bathing and washing of children. *The Trained Nurse, 3*(2), 89–93.

Staggers, N., & Jennings, B. M. (2009). The content and context of change of shift report on medical and surgical units. *Journal of Nursing Administration, 39,* 393–398.

Starker, S. (1978). Case conference and tribal ritual: Some cognitive, social, and anthropologic aspects of the case conference. *Journal of Personality and Social Systems, 1*(4), 3–14.

Stender, I. M., Blichmann, C., & Serup, J. (1990). Effects of oil and water baths on the hydration state of the epidermis. *Clinical and Experimental Dermatology, 15,* 206–209.

Stewart-Amidei, C. (1994). Traditions. *Journal of Neuroscience Nursing, 26,* 259.

Stolzenberger, K. M. (2003). Beyond the Magnet Award: The ANCC program as the framework for culture change. *Journal of Nursing Administration, 33,* 522–531.

Strange, F. (1996). Handover: An ethnographic study of ritual in nursing practice. *Intensive and Critical Care Nursing, 12,* 106–112.

Strange, F. (2001). The persistence of ritual in nursing practice. *Clinical Effectiveness in Nursing, 5,* 177–183. doi: 10.1054/cein.2001.0240

Strauss, A., & Corbin, J. (1998). *Basics of qualitative research: Techniques and procedures for developing grounded theory.* London, UK: Sage.

Strople, B., & Ottani, P. (2006). Can technology improve intershift report? What research reveals. *Journal of Professional Nursing, 22,* 197–204.

Suominen, T., Kovasin, M., & Ketola, O. (1997). Nursing culture: Some viewpoints. *Journal of Advanced Nursing, 25,* 186–190.

Swanson, K. M. (1991). Empirical development of a middle range theory of caring. *Nursing Research, 40,* 161–166.

Swanson, K. M. (1999). What's known about caring in nursing: A literary meta-analysis. In A. S. Hinshaw, J. Shaver, & S. Feetham (Eds.), *Handbook of clinical nursing research* (pp. 31–60). Thousand Oaks, CA: Sage.

Taft, L. (2005). Apology and medical mistake: Opportunity or foil? *Annals of Health Law, 14,* 55–94.

Talcott, S. H. (1895). A lecture on cleanliness. *The Trained Nurse, 14*, 31.

Tambia, J. (1968). The magical power of words. *Man, 3*, 175–208.

Taxis, K., & Barber, N. (2003). Causes of intravenous medication errors: An ethnographic study. *Quality and Safety in Health Care, 12*, 343–347. Retrieved from ProQuest Central.

Taylor, B. J. (1994). *Being human: Ordinariness in nursing*. Melbourne, Australia: Churchill Livingstone.

Tejero, L. M. S. (2011). The mediating role of the nurse–patient dyad bonding in bringing about patient satisfaction. *Journal of Advanced Nursing, 68*, 994–1002. doi: 10.1111/j.1365 -2648.2011.05795.x

Terry (2007). Triple check that medication vial! *Nursing Voices Forum*. Retrieved from http:// www.nursingvoices.com/general-nursing-topics/25-triple-check-medication-vial.html

Thomson, H. (2009). Stop the slide in standards of care with some sound basic procedures. *Nursing Standard, 24*(18), 24.

Thornby, D. (2006). Beginning the journey to skilled communication. *AACN Advanced Critical Care, 17*, 266–271.

Thorne, S., & Paterson, B. (1998). Shifting images of chronic illness. *Image: Journal of Nursing Scholarship, 30*, 173–178.

Timmermans, S. (2005). Death brokering: Constructing culturally appropriate death. *Sociology of Health & Illness, 27*, 993–1013. doi: 10.1111/j.1467-9566.2005.00467.x

Tissot, E., Cornette, C., Demoly, P., Jacquet, M., Barale, F., & Capelier, G. (1999). Medication errors at the administration stage in an intensive care unit. *Intensive Care Medicine, 25*, 353–359.

Tonuma, M., & Winbolt, M. (2000). From rituals to reason: Creating an environment that allows nurses to nurse. *International Journal of Nursing Practice, 6*, 214–218.

Touhy, T. (1997). The complexity of basic care. *Journal of Gerontological Nursing, 23*(5), 5–6.

Treiber, L. A., & Jones, J. H. (2010). Devastatingly human: An analysis of registered nurses' medication error accounts. *Qualitative Health Research, 20*, 1327–1342. doi: 10.1177/1049732310372228

Tudor, J. (1890). After death. *The Trained Nurse, 5*, 225–226.

Turner, E. (1992). *Experiencing ritual*. Philadelphia, PA: University of Pennsylvania Press.

Turner, V. (1967). *The forest of symbols. Aspects of Ndembu ritual*. New York, NY: Cornell University Press.

Turner, V. (1969). *The ritual process: Structure and anti-structure*. Ithaca, NY: Cornell University Press.

Turner, V. (1974). *Dramas, fields, and metaphors: Symbolic action in human society*. Ithaca, NY: Cornell University Press.

Twigg, J. (2000). Carework as a form of bodywork. *Aging and Society, 20*, 389–411.

Twigg, J. (2002). The body in social policy: Mapping a territory. *Journal of Social Policy, 31*, 421–439. doi: 10.1017/S0047279402006645

Tyndale, W. (1992). *Tyndale's Old Testament*. New Haven, CT: Yale University Press.

University of Oklahoma, School of Nursing. (1951). Striping Ceremony, Program, Robert M. Bird Health Sciences Library. Nursing_Box41_20110419_141948. Retrieved from http: //birdlibrary.contentdm.oclc.org/cdm/landingpage/collection/p15191coll3

U.S. Department of Defense. (n.d.). *Briefs and huddles toolkit*. Retrieved from http://health .mil/dodpatientsafety/ProductsandServices/Toolkits/BriefsHuddles.aspx

U.S. Fed News Service, Including U.S. State News. (2012). Nursing pinning ceremony 2012. Retrieved from ProQuest Central: http://dbproxy.lasalle.edu:4332/docview/10157 82648?accountid=11999

van Gennep, A. (1960). *The rites of passage*. Chicago, IL: University of Chicago Press.

Van Manen, M. (1990). *Researching lived experience: Human science for an action sensitive peda-gogy*. New York, NY: State University of New York Press.

Veterans Affairs Maryland Health Care System. (2012, May 12). VA Maryland Health Care System observes Nurses Week with awards ceremony. Retrieved from prweb, http://www.redorbit.com/news/health/1112528934/va_maryland_health_care_system_observes_nurses_week_with_awards

Villanueva, N. E. (1999). Experiences of critical care nurses caring for unresponsive patients. *Journal of Neuroscience Nursing, 31,* 200–257.

Wagnild, G., & Manning, R. W. (1985). Convey respect during bathing procedures. *Journal of Gerontological Nursing, 11*(12), 6–10.

Walker, V. (1967). *Nursing and ritualistic practice.* New York, NY: Macmillan.

Walsh, M., & Ford, P. (1989). Rituals in nursing: "We always do it this way." *Nursing Times, 85*(41), 35.

Walter, T. (2003). Hospices and rituals after death: A survey of British hospice chaplains. *International Journal of Hospice Care, 9,* 80–85.

Ward, L. (2010). Care after death. *Nursing Standard, 25*(13), 59.

Watson Caring Science Institute. (n.d.). Caring science (Definitions, processes, theory: Transpersonal caring and the caring moment defined. Retrieved from http://watsoncaringscience.org/about-us/caring-science-definitions-processes-theory/

Watson, J. (1988). New dimensions of Human Caring Theory. *Nursing Science Quarterly, 1,* 175–181. doi: 10.1177/089431848800100411

Watson, J. (1999). *Postmodern nursing and beyond.* Toronto, Canada: Churchill Livingstone.

Watson, J. (2001). Jean Watson: Theory of human caring. In M. E. Parker (Ed.), *Nursing theories and nursing practice* (pp. 343–354). Philadelphia, PA: F. A. Davis.

Watson, J. (2002). Intentionality and caring-healing consciousness: A practice of transpersonal nursing. *Holistic Nursing Practice, 16*(4), 12–19.

Watson, J. (2005). *Caring science as sacred science.* Philadelphia, PA: F. A. Davis.

Watson, J. (2006). Caring theory as an ethical guide to administrative and clinical practices. *Nursing Science Quarterly, 30*(1), 48–55.

Watson, J. (n.d.). *Transpersonal caring and the caring moment defined.* Retrieved from http://watsoncaringscience.org/about-us/caring-science-definitions-processes-theory/

Watson Caring Science Institute. (2010). Core concepts of Jean Watson's Theory of Human Caring/caring science. Retrieved from http://mercycadillac.munsonhealthcare.org/munson/health_education/classes_programs/ictp-handouts/1a-CoreConcepts.pdf

Watson Caring Science Institute. (n.d.). Caring Science Ten Caritas Processes: Transpersonal Caring and the Caring Moment Defined. Retrieved from http://www.watsoncaringscience.org/index.cfm/category/80/theory.cfm#

"What happened to the cap?" (n.d.). Retrieved from http://justusnurses.com/forum/f155/what-happened-cap-7635

While, A., & Dewsbury, G. (2011). Nursing and information and communication technology (ICT): A discussion of trends and future directions. *International Journal of Nursing Studies, 48,* 1302–1310.

Wilson, B. (2006). Pre-pouring medications. *Nursing BC, 38*(2), 9.

Wilson, D., & DiVito-Thomas, P. (2004). The sixth right of medication administration. Right response. *Nurse Educator, 29,* 131–132.

Wilson, J., Thompson-Hill, J., & Chaplin, D. (2010). National guidance on last offices would prevent family distress. *Nursing Times, 106*(27), 8.

Winkelstein, M. L., Huss, K., Butz, A., Eggleston, P., Vargas, P., & Rand, C. (2000). Factors associated with medication self-administration in children with asthma. *Clinical Pediatrics, 39,* 337–345.

Winsett, R. P., & Hauck, S. (2011). Implementing relationship-based care. *Journal of Nursing Administration, 41,* 285–290.

Winslow, E. H., Lane, L. D., & Gaffney, F. A. (1985). Oxygen uptake and cardiovascular responses in control adults and acute myocardial infarction patients during bathing. *Nursing Resarch, 34,* 164–169.

Wolf, Z. R. (1986a). *Nursing rituals in an adult acute care hospital: An ethnography.* Ann Arbor, MI: University Microfilms.

Wolf, Z. R. (1986b). Nurses' work: The sacred and the profane. *Holistic Nursing Practice, 1*(1), 29–33.

Wolf, Z. R. (1988a). *Nurses' work: The sacred and the profane.* Philadelphia, PA: University of Pennsylvania Press.

Wolf, Z. R. (1988b). Nursing rituals. *Canadian Journal of Nursing Research, 20*(3), 59–69.

Wolf, Z. R. (1989a). Uncovering the hidden work of nursing. *Nursing & Health Care, 10,* 463–467.

Wolf, Z. R. (1989b). Medication errors and nursing responsibility. *Holistic Nursing Practice, 4*(1), 8–17.

Wolf, Z. R. (1989c). Learning the professional jargon of nursing during change of shift report. *Holistic Nursing Practice, 4*(1), 78–83.

Wolf, Z. R. (1991a). Care of dying patients and patients after death: Patterns of care in nursing history. *Death Studies, 15,* 81–93.

Wolf, Z. R. (1991b). Nurses' experiences giving postmortem care to patients who have donated organs: A phenomenological study. *Scholarly Inquiry for Nursing Practice: An International Journal, 5*(2), 73–87.

Wolf, Z. R. (1993). The bath: A nursing ritual. *Journal of Holistic Nursing, 11,* 135–148.

Wolf, Z. R. (1994). *Medication errors: The nursing experience.* New York, NY: Delmar.

Wolf, Z. R. (1997). Nursing students' experience bathing patients for the first time. *Nurse Educator, 22*(2), 41–46.

Wolf, Z. R. (2007). Pursuing safe medication use and the promise of technology. *MEDSURG Nursing, 16*(2), 92–100.

Wolf, Z. R. (2009). Knowing patients' bodies: Nurses' bodywork. In R. C. Locsin & M. J. Purnell (Eds.), *A contemporary nursing process: The (un)bearable weight of knowing in nursing* (pp. 177–203). New York, NY: Springer.

Wolf, Z. R. (2010). Clinical nurse specialists and difficult clinician–patient situations: Strategies for success. In P. R. Zuzelo (Ed.), *Clinical nurse specialist workbook* (2nd ed., pp. 147–181). Sudbury, MA: Jones & Bartlett.

Wolf, Z. R., & Hughes, R. G. (2008). Error reporting and error disclosure. In R. Hughes (Ed.). *Healthcare error book* (chap. 35). Rockville, MD: Agency for Healthcare Research and Quality.

Wolf, Z. R., & Robinson-Smith, G. (2007). Strategies used by clinical nurse specialist to care for "difficult" clinician–ptaient situations: A descriptive study. *Clinical Nurse Specialist, 21*(2), 74–84.

Wolf, Z. R., Serembus, J. F., & Youngblood, N. (2001). Consequences of fatal medication errors for health care providers: A secondary analysis study. *MEDSURG Nursing, 10*(4), 193–201.

Wolf, Z. R., & Smith, P. A. (1997). Direct and indirect care: Defining domains of nursing practice. *International Journal for Human Caring, 1*(3), 43–52.

Wooten, N. (2000). Evaluation of 12-hour shifts on a cardiology nursing development unit. *British Journal of Nursing, 9,* 2169–2174.

Wright, K. (2005). Unsupervised medication administration by nursing students. *Nursing Standard, 19*(3), 49–54. Retrieved from ProQuest Central.

Yonge, O. (2008). Shift report: A ritual play on a residential adolescent psychiatric unit. *Journal of Psychiatric and Mental Health Nursing, 15,* 45–51.

Yoshino, R. (1993). Magical numbers of human short-term memory: Efficient designs of biological memory systems? *Behaviormetrika, 20,* 171–186.

Zimmerman, P. G. (2006). Cutting-edge discussions of management, policy, and program issues in emergency care. *Journal of Emergency Nursing, 32,* 178–185.

INDEX